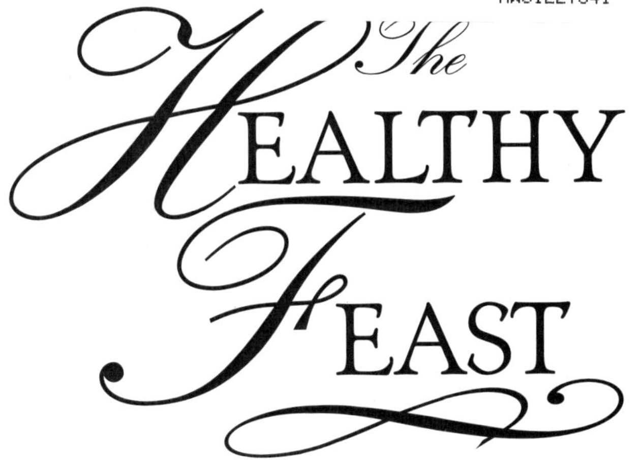

The Healthy Feast

Cooking Light with Mediterranean Oils

Mark Emmerson

and

Jeannette Ewin, Ph.D.

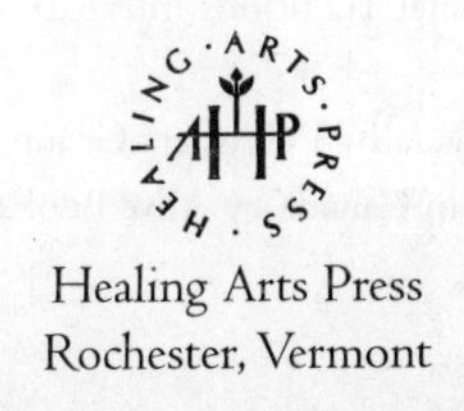

Healing Arts Press
Rochester, Vermont

Healing Arts Press
One Park Street
Rochester, Vermont 05767
www.gotoit.com

This Healing Arts Press edition published in agreement with Thorsons, an imprint of HarperCollins*Publishers,* 1997

First published under the title *A Feast of Oils* by Thorsons 1996

Note to the reader: This book is intended as an informational guide. The remedies, approaches, and techniques described herein are meant to supplement, and not to be a substitute for, professional medical care or treatment. They should not be used to treat a serious ailment without prior consultation with a qualified health-care professional.

Library of Congress Cataloging-in-Publication Data
Emmerson, Mark.
The healthy feast : cooking light with Mediterranean oils / Mark Emmerson and Jeannette Ewin.
p. cm.
Originally published: A feast of oils. London : Thorsons, 1996.
Includes bibliographical references (p.) and index.
ISBN 0-89281-742-9
1. Oils and fats, Edible. 2. Low-fat diet—Recipes. I. Ewin, Jeannette. II. Ewin, Jeannette. Feast of oils. III. Title.
TX407.034E55 1997 97-22872
641.5'638—dc21 CIP

Printed and bound in the United States

10 9 8 7 6 5 4 3 2 1

Illustrations by Laila Brieze

Healing Arts Press is a division of Inner Traditions International

Distributed to the book trade in Canada by Publishers Group West (PGW), Toronto, Ontario
Distributed to the health food trade in Canada by Alive Books, Toronto and Vancouver

For Nicole and Richard

Acknowledgements

Inspiration for this book came from many people. In particular, Jeannette and I thank Charles and Sika Cary, owners of The Oil Merchant, and Tony Greenwood, from Selfridges Food Hall, for their expert advice. Also, Wanda Whiteley, our Senior Editor at Thorsons, for supporting our ideas and encouraging us throughout the writing of this book, Michelle Clark, who patiently edited the manuscript, and all the people at HarperCollins who took our words and made them into a beautiful book. Above all, however, I personally want to thank Peter Kromberg, Chef at Le Soufflé, London, who inspired me to become a dedicated chef, and who has always been there for me throughout my career.

Mark Emmerson

Contents

List of Recipes

Preface

This book contains more than just recipes – it introduces a new way of thinking about food, and it could change the way you cook forever. By preparing and keeping a few special oils and oil-based ingredients on hand, you can make delicious foods and dramatically reduce the amount of saturated fat in your diet.

In the next few chapters, you will learn how the various oils differ, how to balance their flavours with other ingredients and why they offer a totally new way to keep the foods you prepare light and healthy. Because the demand for oils has increased dramatically over the past decade, dozens of varieties are widely available – from a most wonderful, international assortment of fine virgin olive oils to a vast range of less commonly used unrefined nut oils, such as walnut, hazelnut and almond. Their tastes are exciting and they broaden the scope of healthy foods you can prepare at home.

By using the recipes given here, you can enjoy flavour-packed dishes that look marvellous and are rich in nutritional goodness. As a bonus, once you learn to make the basic ingredients – the foundation recipes given in Chapter 2 – preparing food for both family and friends will be faster, easier and much more fun.

Some of these recipes are ideal for quick snacks. Deep-fried Root Vegetables, for example, are easy-to-make treats that double-up as a scrumptious savoury garnish. Other dishes are splendid, easy-to-prepare party pieces. You need never tell your guests just how simple it is to make Chinese-style Monkfish Ravioli or a perfect plate of Crispy-skinned Wild Salmon with Rice Noodles.

Be warned: this is not a book about substituting a splash of oil for a chunk of butter in a frying pan. Learning the proper way to cook with oils calls for a little time and experimentation. Here you will find out about tasting, blending and savouring the distinctive characters and aromas of oils – not just any oils, but fine oils with qualities as complicated and rewarding as those enjoyed in good wine. Because this book is about getting to know and enjoy a new style of cooking, spend some time browsing through the first two chapters and thinking about how the ideas suggested can be adapted to your kitchen.

Chapter 1, The basics – selecting and enjoying oils, explains how to select, store and use oils. Chapter 2, The foundation recipes, describes methods for making your own infusions, including one that captures the dark flavours of wild mushrooms and another that shelters the aromatic gold of saffron. Both are excellent ingredients that enhance foods as different as risotto and polenta. By mastering the other basic foundation recipes, you will soon be making your own black olive tapenade, succulent oven-dried tomatoes, pistou and delicious fennel stock.

Many of the recipes in Chapter 3, Recipes for healthy eating, are adaptations of dishes we serve at the restaurant, One Paston Place. Guests may recognize the simple – but popular – Crushed Potato with Spring Onions (Scallions) and Flat-leaf Parsley (Italian Parsley), and the Polenta with Grilled (Broiled) Asparagus and Wild Mushrooms. What they may not have appreciated until now, however, is just how low in saturated fats these favourites really are. In some cases the methods for the recipes are detailed, but don't be daunted as they are there to explain certain important techniques as clearly as possible to ensure success, such as cleaning artichokes and double-frying mushrooms.

There was a time when I used a considerable amount of butter and cream in my cooking. Then I discovered how delicious and light foods prepared with oils can be. Soon, butter and cream almost vanished from our kitchen. Today, when Skinless Grilled (Broiled) Chicken Breast with Mushroom Tapenade and Savoy Cabbage appears on the menu, I know our guests will enjoy beautiful, healthy food with real flavour value.

My goal in cooking is to prepare food that is enjoyable to look at and taste, but is also nutritious. When selecting the recipes for this book, I did so with this aim in mind. As a result, you will find only one case where cream is mentioned – and that is as an alternative ingredient. No butter is used, nor is there any need for beef or rich lamb.

It is more than the oils alone that make these recipes suitable for healthy eating, it is the fresh vegetables and a variety of fish that contribute too. Some of the dishes are ideal for vegetarians, while others for meat eaters feature light meats, such as chicken breast, duck and quail. Marvellous fish – such as fresh tuna, salmon and mackerel – are prepared in ways that bring out the best in their texture and flavour. Hot-smoking, marinades and grilling (broiling) techniques add diversity to the ways in which these oily fish can be served. I have included a number of fish recipes here because of the health benefits we can derive from the precious omega–3 essential fatty acids they contain.

Another important feature of this book is the Afterword. Most people are surprised when I tell them there are fats they *need* to eat. The Afterword, therefore, is required reading because, in a series of answers to basic questions about dietary fats, you learn how and why cooking with oils will not only heighten the flavour and quality of what you prepare, but add years to your life and a spring to your step.

During the past few years, scientists, politicians and, yes, even food writers, have stressed the dangers in what we eat. We believe that puts things the wrong way around. Food is our friend; it is the stuff of life and good health, and one of the most enjoyable aspects of living. While we obviously agree that sensible choices are best, we also encourage you to fully enjoy the experience of what you cook and eat. Smell, feel, and, most of all, appreciate the tastes of the great international mixture of foods available today. As a part of that experience, we hope this book will help you enjoy a feast of oils.

Mark Emmerson and Jeannette Ewin

The Basics – Selecting and Enjoying Oils

Some dull facts about a splendid food – oil

A speedy review of some rudimentary biology helps explain the reasons for cooking with oils. Proteins, carbohydrates, an assortment of vitamins and minerals and fats combine to form all living things. For normal growth and good health, a proper balance of all these substances must be obtained from the foods we eat, including fats.

Saturated fats are stiff, or inflexible, and fats rich in these molecules tend to be solids at room temperature or below. That is why the fat left on a plate after a steak dinner becomes hard when cool. Unsaturated fats, on the other hand, bend, they are flexible, thus forming oils at room temperature. Saturated fats store food energy, but have no other unique nutritional value. Unsaturated fats, however, are needed for normal growth and good health because they include certain specific fatty acids known as *essential fatty acids*. These substances cannot be manufactured by the human body and so must be part of the foods we eat. That is why we should eat fewer saturated fats and more unsaturated fats, like those found in oils.

The links between fats, health and diet are discussed further in the Afterword.

So, what is an 'extra virgin' oil?

Deciphering food labels is difficult at best, but with oils, some of the 'cuisine babble' is almost beyond comprehension. As a rule of thumb, though, terms used to describe oils reflect the extent to which they are processed. To remove the first veil of confusion, let us separate terms used for nut and seed oils from the more romantic labels used for olive oil.

Oil in nuts and seeds may be separated from their pulp by pressure, but the yield is small and fat-soluble natural substances are carried into the oil. As a result, these *unrefined* oils maintain the distinctive colour and flavour of the nut or seed and so are ideal for many of the recipes in this book. Oils containing these substances, and sometimes bits of pulp, carry the richest colour and flavour of the original seed or nut, making them ideal for certain purposes. Because the minimum amount has been done to extract the oil, it is called *unrefined,* and because the yield is low, the cost per unit volume will be high. However, the same substances that give these oils their special qualities also make them susceptible to damage by heat and exposure to the air, so they are best for flavouring salads and sauces and should not be used for frying. Unrefined olive oils are also known as extra virgin oils, or *first pressing*.

To increase the yield from seeds and nuts, and reduce the unit cost of the product, manufacturers use more intensive extraction methods. They may increase the pressure (and generate heat in the process) or combine heat and pressure in the pressing process or they may employ a chemical extraction process. The oils that result from these manufacturing processes are clean and contain none of the bits of natural debris and only very modest amounts of the natural non-oily substances that give unrefined oils their character. However, these *refined* oils are excellent foods because they are lower in cost, have a longer shelf-life and a greater capacity to withstand heat in cooking and the manufacture of other products.

Some fine nut oils are produced by pressing with light heat. Toasted almond oil and roasted peanut oil are two that come to mind. Walnut oil, which is highly nutritious, has been popular in various regions of France for centuries as a cooking ingredient in sauces and dressings. However, it goes rancid quickly and so is usually purchased in small quantities. Such oils are definitely still worth buying as they add much to the enjoyment of food.

Olive oil is not obtained from the seed or nut of a plant, but from its oil-rich fruit. For centuries, olive oil has been produced by gently pressing a pulp of crushed olives. The first oil collected for eating is dark green and highly flavoured; this is the *extra virgin* oil and is the most expensive. The pulp is then re-pressed, using greater force, to produce a slightly lesser grade – *virgin* oil. After that, if heat and/or chemical means are used to increase the total yield from the pulp, *refined* oils are produced. The later an oil is obtained in this extraction process, the lighter its colour and flavour. To some tastes, the more processed, or refined, olive oils are more desirable because they are not dominated by the taste of the fruit. To others, the characteristic flavours and aroma of extra virgin oils justify a handsome price.

Like fine wines, the flavour and colour of olive oils are affected by the location in which the fruit is grown. Temperature, rainfall and the quality of the soil all influence the green-gold liquids that form handsome displays in markets, food halls and speciality shops.

For more information about specific oils, see the Directory of Cooking Oils, at the back of this book.

Tasting oils

Variety is one of the reasons I enjoy cooking with oils. Exploring the many tastes, colours, weights and characteristics of new oils is as exciting and rewarding as trying a selection of vintage wines. When my suppliers offer a new oil, whether it is virgin olive oil from a new estate or a hazelnut oil from a new source, it deserves careful and slow assessment before I decide whether or not to add it to my collection.

When you begin using oils as a major ingredient in cooking, it is important to try enough varieties to get to know which you personally prefer. I have used the analogy already, but, it is so apt – in many ways, tasting oils is like tasting wines, although I suggest swallowing them rather than spitting them out! And, as with wines, don't be afraid to try oil 'straight'. After all, enjoying a drink of pure olive oil, as if it were a fine whisky, is an everyday occurrence for many people living in the sun-drenched areas around the Mediterranean Sea.

The finest oils are expensive, however. A half-litre bottle of the best-quality walnut oil will cost as much as a bottle of vintage port, so it should be treated with respect. To make it a little more affordable, I suggest you ask a local speciality food shop to set up a tasting for you or, alternatively, share the enjoyment with some friends and split the costs.

You judge fine things – whether it is wine, a sauce or vinegars and oils – on their character. That is what it is all about. If you taste something and think, 'Oh, that is very nice' and two seconds later you have nothing left in your mouth, then that dish has no character. Character is what you want in top-quality oils.

How do you judge the character of an oil? First and foremost, by its flavour, but, before you get to that point, you need to evaluate how you like its colour (that will affect how you combine it with other foods), its aroma and the weight it has in your mouth. Some oils leave a soft sensation on the tongue; others make it feel rather furry.

To sample oils, I suggest you use coffee cups. I prefer the sensation of china rather than glass while I'm tasting oil, but it is a matter of personal choice. Pour a small amount (a tablespoon at most) into the cup and swirl it around. First, see how you like the colour on the cup, then sniff it, taking a good noseful of its aroma. For some oils, you may find you want to stop there! Some roasted nut oils can be overpowering.

While you are evaluating the aroma, think which foods could benefit from this particular oil. Are they foods your family enjoys?

Next, taste the oil. This is a good place to stop and jot down your impressions. Then, before you go on to the next oil, eat a small piece of bread or some other neutral food to cleanse your mouth before you try the next oil on offer. Some cookery experts suggest dipping bread into the oil before tasting it, but I do not see the point in this, as the aroma and texture of the bread interferes with the sensations you are receiving from the oil.

Finally, once you find one or two oils you prefer, do not splash out on the large, economy-sized bottles; buy in small quantities – quality depends on freshness.

What goes with what?

Different oils dominate different cuisines around the world. Sesame and soya feature in dishes from Asia and the Middle East, corn oil in those from America, olive oil those from Europe and mustard oil those from India. These oils tell us something about the plants indigenous to these areas and also explain why foods from specific regions have characteristic flavours.

When deciding which oils you will use to build your own collection, think about the typical foods from these regions, the tastes of the oils used and types of ingredients used in dishes from the regions. Indeed, this is a good place to begin thinking about combining oils with foods in your own kitchen. Olive oil blends well with the basic texture and taste of pasta for example, whereas you might find mustard oil unappetizing in the same dish. Similarly, sesame oil is delicious with oriental vegetables and rice, but would not be an ideal choice for a tomato and basil salad. For fish, neutral oils – such as sunflower and grapeseed – add texture but do not detract from the flavour of the fish, which is why they are the right choice for many fish marinades.

Experiment with oils by themselves before you combine them with other ingredients. Try dark, rich nut oils with pâtés and meat salads. For example, spoon a few drops of unrefined nut oil around a plate of duck liver pâté – pistachio oil is excellent for this, if you can find it. A sparing amount of hazelnut oil mixed with mashed parsnips (see page 98) or floated on a plate next to cold meat terrine, will significantly enhance the total flavour and aroma of the dish.

Olives and duck are a combination that has enjoyed success for centuries. A full-flavoured olive oil is a fine complement to a dish made with duck, a salad or may add appeal to a side dish, such as a bowl of finely cut sautéd cabbage. Nut oil, similar to olive oil in smoothness and tone, may also be used for duck or dark-fleshed game birds, such as partridge.

Some of the richer flavoured nut oils, such as walnut and hazelnut, are good partners for densely flavoured red meats – beef, venison and boar, for example. They are also delicious on apple salads and in many desserts. However, flavours can vary. If you are using walnut oil, consider the depth of 'huskiness' in its flavour. These are some of the most exciting oils on the market, but extraction methods will vary the taste. Sometimes some husk is left in place during processing. If there is enough taste of husk to produce a slightly bitter undertone, that particular walnut oil may not be the best choice for anything but the strongest game.

Essential oils

The focus of this book is edible oils, like those obtained from nuts and seeds, but it is worth mentioning essential oils briefly. *Essential fatty acids* are not to be confused with *essential oils*. They are two very different substances and come from totally separate parts of the plant. *Essential fatty acids* are true fats, needed for normal growth and good health. *Essential oils* are highly scented substances that carry the 'essential' aromatic characteristics of the plant. They are not required nutrients, although some have found favour among herbalists for the treatment of certain health conditions and their flavour power has been exploited in the food manufacturing industry for decades.

Some general cooking tips

Before you read the foundation recipes in the next chapter, let me pass on some tips about basic flavours and techniques you can use in all of your cooking. Please don't disregard them because they appear so elementary – little changes make big differences when it comes to bringing out the best in food.

- Use fresh herbs. Disregard what you have read about dried herbs having stronger flavours – they do not. The unique flavours and scents of herbs come from highly aromatic substances that quickly evaporate when their leaves and stems are bruised, dried or heated. Try growing some herbs, such as flat-leaf parsley (Italian parsley), rosemary, thyme, basil and marjoram, in a few pots on your patio or in a corner of the garden. Flat-leaf parsley is a favourite of mine and is included in many of the recipes collected here. It has a wonderful taste, great colour and is packed with beta-carotene – a substance hailed for its ability to fight ageing and disease.

- Use freshly ground black pepper. Pepper is a much underrated spice because it is used so frequently. We forget the distinctive, powerful, aromatic quality of pepper's flavour if we only use the powdery, pre-ground variety from a shaker. Pepper's goodness is locked in its essential, aromatic oils, which are soon lost to the atmosphere. If the peppercorns are ground, or crushed, just before serving, the maximum flavour is transferred to the food we are about to enjoy. (If you want the taste of black pepper, but not the hard black bits, make an oil infusion. Pour crushed black peppercorns into a bottle of oil and let it stand for at least two days before using. Choose an oil with little flavour of its own – sunflower for example.)
- Use non-stick cooking utensils whenever you can, but purchase the heavy grade variety as they last longer and withstand heat better. Non-stick pans allow you to fry and crisp foods using only a very modest amount of fat.
- Consider what a plate of food will look like before you begin cooking. Plan how you are going to ensure variations of colour and texture of the ingredients you want to combine in a dish. For example, garnishing the finished dish is always worth while, whereas serving white fish with mashed potatoes and sautéd parsnips will mean setting an insipid-looking plate on the table. Consider steamed broccoli instead and a garnish of oven-dried tomatoes or a spicy red vinaigrette over the fish.
- Quality matters. Use fresh, prime ingredients in the foods you prepare, especially when you are cooking fish and poultry. It is better to buy a modest amount of a prime ingredient, than to purchase a larger quantity of a lesser quality product. The latter will not produce the same fine eating experience. It is a false economy.

One final thought: food is about life, and life is about sharing. Cook for health, but also cook for the pleasure of breaking bread with family and friends.

The Foundation Recipes

Let's get started! Here are the foundation, or basic, recipes that introduce you to lighter, easier cooking. They contain no saturated fats and provide a range of textures and flavours you can use time and again in your cooking. Some of these recipes are excellent on their own, as snacks; others are best blended with other ingredients for maximum appeal. Although you will find suggestions with each on how they can be used, you will soon adapt these to meet your own likes and dislikes. Just as an artist knows which colours to choose when painting a sunset or misty harbour scene, a good cook knows which basic recipes give the flavour, depth and texture needed in a specific dish.

How to ensure success

Always measure the quantities of ingredients given in the recipes carefully using a good kitchen scale and proper measuring spoons (and cup measures), filling them until they are level. Do not mix the metric, imperial and American measures in the same recipe as they are not interchangeable. All the recipes give metric measures first with imperial and American equivalents in brackets – imperial first, American second.

Do follow the list of ingredients and methods given closely as sometimes even the simplest change can ruin what would otherwise have been a successful dish. A poorly balanced vinaigrette, an oxidized infusion or a curdled mayonnaise will detract from good food as much as will a bad bottle of wine.

Making infusions

An *infusion* is a fluid that has taken up the flavour and scent of another substance. Wines can be infused with cloves and nutmeg, milk with vanilla pods (beans) and water with tea. Oils make excellent infusions because they absorb and hold flavours and colours that are soluble in fats.

Natural plant flavours – for example those found in the skins of lemons or basil leaves – most often occur in the form of terpenes, which are small, fat-soluble molecules. These are not easily transferred to water or wine and deteriorate quickly once a transfer has been achieved. By contrast, the distinctive flavours and colours of specific plants can last for weeks in oil when stored under the right conditions. The earthy characteristics of black truffles, for example, are soon lost when they are infused into wine, but will last for months in a well-cared-for bottle of virgin olive oil.

In part, this is because natural substances found in oils – such as the powerful antioxidant, vitamin E – protect the blend of oil and plant molecules from becoming rancid (oxidized) and decomposing. Processed oils, including the blended vegetable oils available for deep frying, can be used as the base for an infusion, but they contain fewer natural protective substances than virgin olive oil. They also have little of their own character to add to the final product.

The flavour and colour of the oil you choose for an infusion establishes the base for what is to come. If it has a natural green tone – as you will find in a fine, dark green pistachio oil – it may not be a good choice for an infusion you are planning to use on white fish. A brown walnut oil may look right with mushrooms, but all wrong on steamed cauliflower. Equally, if an oil has a heavy taste of olives, it may be all wrong for fruity infusions – say one made with tangerine peel. In such a case, a neutral oil, such as sunflower, would be best as it would add little colour or taste to the final product. Alternatively, a heady, unrefined virgin olive oil – from Tuscany, for example – will lend its own flavour and aroma to a mixture, making it an ideal base for a hearty infusion of herbs and garlic.

Most oil infusions are simple and highly rewarding to make. In the dead of winter, when the herbs in your garden have disappeared, what better way to lift your spirits and cooking than by opening a bottle of infused oil you made the previous summer? Savour its aroma and think of warm days as you decant a quantity over a portion of poached fish or toss a few drops into a green salad.

General tips for making oil infusions

- Make certain your containers are clean and dry before use. There are a number of ways to sterilize containers. One of the easiest is to wash and dry them in a dishwasher. Another is to wash them in hot, soapy water and rinse them well with boiling water. Alternatively, wash them, top up with water and allow them to stand in a medium oven until the water begins to 'move' in the container, then leave them to cool, empty them and allow them to air dry.
- Consider how much oil you plan to use and choose container sizes accordingly. Because oxidization – rancidity – is always a problem when using oils, smaller rather than larger containers are often best.
- Ceramic and glazed pottery containers may be used, but glass is best because it withstands the high temperatures needed for sterilization. Also, it will add no flavour of its own – a problem with some glazed clay containers such as those sometimes used for marinating olives.
- Choose containers with a good lid or seal. Air and air-born bacteria can ruin your efforts.
- Use high-quality oils, herbs and spices because, as is true in all cooking, the final product will be no better than the ingredients used. Peppercorns, cloves and cinnamon, for example, should be freshly purchased, not ones you have had standing in an opened bottle on the shelf for a year.
- Wash herbs and press them dry with paper kitchen towel to remove any extra moisture. Moisture will cloud and destroy the quality of the infusion.
- Brushing or bruising hard herbs (thyme, rosemary and sage, for example) helps release their flavours into the oil. Soft herbs, such as basil, chervil and tarragon, require no prior treatment except cleaning.
- Plan ahead. Allow adequate time for flavours to infuse.
- When using herbs – parsley, mint, basil and chervil, for example – use the best and freshest you can find. Avoid the temptation to pour a packet of dried herbs into a bottle of oil; they will fail to give off a good flavour or colour. Drying does not concentrate the natural flavour and colour of herbs; its effects are quite the opposite.
- If you wish to use fresh garlic, red pepper (bell pepper) or onions – all of which have a high water content – make certain you keep your infusion in the refrigerator and use it within two to three weeks. Water contained in the ingredients will speed deterioration and cause the infusion to become cloudy. When an infusion clouds, make a fresh batch. (The one exception to this rule involves certain olive oils, which cloud in cool temperatures because

of their high monounsaturated fatty acid content. When using olive oil, check its appearance after a few hours in the refrigerator to get an idea of its normal appearance.)

- After an infusion has 'matured' for at least two weeks, the oil can be strained into another clean container. A funnel lined with a clean piece of muslin (cheesecloth) or folded gauze will aid this process.
- Respect garlic and chilli peppers; they are powerful ingredients and can easily overwhelm more delicate flavours.

Making cold infusions

The soft herbs, which include basil, parsley, mint and coriander, add greatly to the taste of many foods. Infusions are an excellent means of introducing their flavour without changing the appearance or cooking characteristics of a dish by the presence of the herb itself.

Two cold infusion methods are popular:

- stuff a sterile glass container with washed and well-dried leaves that have been gently bruised, then fill with oil (make certain the oil covers the top of the leaves and all air is tapped out of the container) and leave in the refrigerator for two weeks, filter and use
- pour some oil into a blender, add one or two handfuls of prepared herbs and blend, then pour the mixture into a prepared container, top up with oil and place in the refrigerator for one or two weeks (when this time has passed, then strain the oil into another sterile, dry container).

'Hard', woody stemmed herbs – such as thyme and rosemary – and fruit peel can also be used in cold infusions. First, wash and dry the ingredient(s) from which you wish to extract the flavour. Second, select an oil. Neutral oils, such as safflower and grapeseed, work well. Third, chop the ingredient(s) coarsely by hand or by fast pulses in a blender. Fourth, place them in a container and add the oil. Fifth, leave in a warm place – such as over a very low heat or in a very low oven – for two to three hours. Sixth, remove the chopped pieces by straining the oil into another container. As this method may introduce some water – especially from peel – allow this second container to stand in the refrigerator overnight, then decant the oil into a final container for storage. Keep in the refrigerator and use within a week.

Flat-leaf Parsley (Italian Parsley) Oil

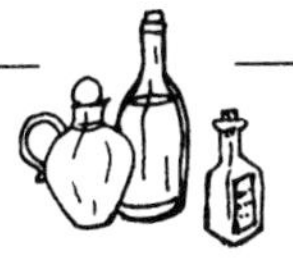

The green colour, light texture and almost neutral flavour of grapeseed oil is perfect for this simple and versatile infusion. If it is not available, try using safflower or sunflower oil. Flat-leaf Parsley (Italian Parsley) Oil is used in several of the recipes in this book: Crispy-skinned Seabass (Striped Bass) with Flat-leaf Parsley (Italian Parsley) and Sorrel Salad (see page 76), and Hot-smoked Fillet of Wild Salmon (see page 78) for example. However, don't limit yourself to my ideas. Once you have made a batch, try some on polenta, on a simple tomato and onion salad, as the base for a mayonnaise or drizzled over a bowl of hot vegetables or whatever else takes your fancy. Its versatile flavour adapts quickly to your personal style of cooking.

Use flat-leaf parsley (Italian parsley) because it has good flavour and colour; curly parsley has less 'oomph'. There is no need to filter Flat-leaf Parsley (Italian Parsley) Oil, but you may wish to do so if you are making a mayonnaise.

This oil can be kept in the refrigerator for one to two weeks.

MAKES 175 ML (6 FL OZ/¾ CUP)

1 bunch (50–75 g/ 2–3 oz) flat-leaf parsley (Italian parsley)
120 ml (4 fl oz/½ cup) grapeseed oil
1 tsp sea salt

1. Pick the leaves off the stalks, then wash and dry them. Put all the ingredients into a blender and blend on full speed for 2 minutes. Then, either use immediately or store for future use in a clean covered jar.

Oil Provençal

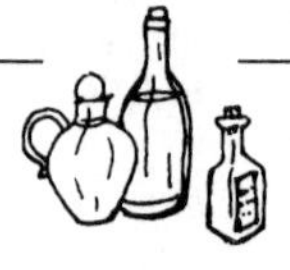

Versatile, simple to make, and saturated with the sun-drenched flavours of southern France, this infusion is another good starting place for experimenting with oils. Try sautéing vegetables in some or drizzle a little over a roasted leg of lamb, lamb cutlets, or on roasted monkfish or use it as a dressing on a salad of roasted vegetables or goat's cheese.

MAKES 500 ML (17 FL OZ/1 GENEROUS US PINT)

2 large sprigs of fresh thyme*
2 large sprigs of fresh rosemary
4 plump cloves of garlic, peeled
500 ml (17 fl oz/1 US pint) extra virgin olive oil

1. Sterilize a 500-ml (17-fl oz/1-US pint) bottle. Make sure it has a tight-fitting lid. Screw-top lids are best, but properly fitted corks are adequate.
2. Bruise the sprigs of thyme and rosemary with the back of a heavy knife. This helps release the flavour from the leaves. Place in the sterilized bottle.
3. Remove the germ** from each garlic clove before adding the clove to the bottle.
4. Top up with good-quality, extra virgin olive oil and screw the lid on. Place in a cool, dark place for at least two weeks, then, once opened, store in the refrigerator.

VARIATION

If you want to make a smaller amount – a quarter or eighth of a litre (8 or 4 fl oz/1 or ½ cup), for example – just push as many herbs as you can into the bottle, plus 1 or 2 cloves of garlic, and top up with virgin olive oil. It's not going to become too overpowering because of the nature of the herbs. If, however, you find your infusion is too strong for your taste, you can always dilute it with extra virgin olive oil.

** What is a large sprig? Try bundling together twigs of rosmary or thyme until they are the thickness of your middle finger. That's about right.*
*** The small green bit of garlic buried in its centre near the bottom end is the germ. It is this part of the clove that makes garlic 'repeat' on many people. Get rid of it by slicing each clove in half lengthwise and sliding out the germ with the tip of a knife.*

Infused Saffron Oil

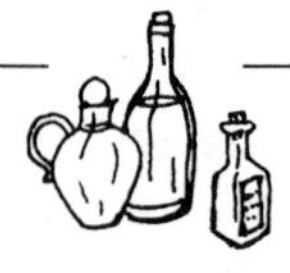

Saffron is an ancient spice that adds greatly to the flavour and colour of many foods, but an expensive one. Each strand of saffron is the stigma from a specific type of crocus flower. The cost of the spice is understandable when you think that each stigma is removed by hand and each 25 g (1 oz) of spice contains between 60 and 70 thousand individual strands. One way to get maximum value from saffron is to capture its colour and flavour in oil.

Saffron oil is excellent as the base for saffron mayonnaise or dripped over baked or grilled (broiled) fish or for flavouring tabboulé or couscous or as the finishing touch for a risotto or – when mashed with roasted garlic and a few drops of balsamic vinegar – as a dip for fresh vegetables.

Stored refrigerated in a covered container, this infusion will keep for two to three weeks.

MAKES 150 ML (5 FL OZ/SCANT ¾ CUP)

150 ml (5 fl oz/generous ½ cup) extra virgin olive oil
2 pieces of dried lemon zest (see below)
2 star anise
1 tsp crushed coriander seeds
1 sprig of thyme
1 tsp sea salt
1 good pinch of saffron strands

1. Place all the ingredients, except the saffron, in a saucepan.
2. Leave, covered, in a cooling but still warm oven (approximately 26°C/80°F) for 2 hours.
3. Strain through muslin (cheesecloth) into a clean bowl or plastic container.
4. Add the saffron strands and, again, leave the oil to infuse in a warm place for 2 hours.

How to Make Lemon Zest

Simply remove strips of rind from untreated, unwaxed lemons with a knife or zester. Place these on a tray in the bottom of a 110°C/225°F/gas ¼ oven for 1–2 hours – until the strips are dry. Then, remove the strips from the oven and store them in a sterilized jar with a tight-fitting lid.

Be sure you use only firm, fresh, untreated lemons, as anything else will give you an inferior product.

Hot infusions

Some ingredients need gentle coaxing before they give up their distinctive flavours and bouquet to oil. Although hot infusions take a bit of time, they are well worth the effort. They concentrate the goodness of ingredients and give extraordinary character to foods. Experiment with the two recipes given here on your family's favourites, as well as the dishes suggested.

While warming oil does damage some of its polyunsaturated goodness, it is still healthier than saturated fats. A tablespoon of Mushroom Oil in risotto, for example, is healthier and gives considerably more character to the dish than a large knob (pat) of butter.

Mushroom Oil

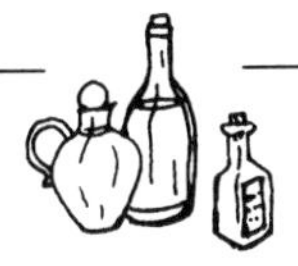

The earthy taste of mushrooms captured in this infusion has a deep richness that maintains its integrity and complements the flavour of most other ingredients. By using Mushroom Oil, rather than mushrooms themselves, you can achieve an excellent aroma and taste without altering the appearance or texture of the foods you add it to.

Mushroom Oil is excellent:

- as a salad dressing (combine some with good-quality balsamic vinegar)
- as a finishing touch in a mushroom sauce or soup
- added to mushroom risotto
- when used to flavour polenta
- combined with garlic and fresh herbs to dress pasta
- drizzled over grilled (broiled) asparagus
- made into mushroom mayonnaise
- combined with Mushroom Tapenade (see page 41) and spread over hot, freshly baked bread.

Choose mushrooms that have depth of flavour. Commercially grown flat field mushrooms are probably the most readily available and least costly flavourful mushrooms, but shiitake mushrooms and French ceps both give excellent results. When available, wild mushrooms also make a fine infusion.

This infusion keeps in the refrigerator for two to three weeks.

MAKES 450 ML (15 FL OZ/SCANT 1 US PINT)

1.5 kg (3 lbs) fresh flat field mushrooms
50 g (2 oz/½ cup) shallots
300 ml (10 fl oz/1¼ cups) grapeseed oil
1 sprig of fresh thyme
2 sprigs of fresh flat-leaf parsley (Italian parsley)
150 ml (5 fl oz/scant ¾ cup) extra virgin olive oil
approximately 1 tsp sea salt

1. Preheat the oven to 110°C/225°F/gas ¼.
2. Brush and wipe the mushrooms free of any debris,* then spread them over a baking sheet in a single layer. Place in the preheated oven for approximately 2 hours, or until the mushrooms are almost brittle. Remove the mushrooms from the oven and leave to cool. Break or tear the mushrooms into pieces.
3. Peel and slice the shallots, put the slices into a deep pan and cook over a low heat in a tablespoon of the grapeseed oil. Add the herbs and dried mushrooms, cook for another 2–3 minutes, then add the remaining grapeseed and the olive oil. Leave to infuse over a very low heat for 1 hour.
4. Pass the oil through a strainer, pressing the mushrooms down with the back of a wooden spoon to extract all the oil. Leave to cool. Store in a clean, tightly capped bottle.

** Do not wash the mushrooms, but brush off any growing media or other matter clinging to them. A piece of paper kitchen towel will do the job very well, but you may enjoy using a mushroom brush, which is specially designed for this purpose.*

Langoustine Oil

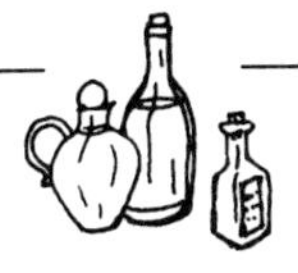

Here is a recipe for gourmets. It takes time, patience and calls for some expensive ingredients, but the impact of its clear, brilliant orange colour and the deep flavour is so powerful that the effort is definitely worth while.

One word concerning nutrition. Because this infusion is heated, it loses some of the health benefits associated with polyunsaturated oil. Nevertheless, because a small amount of Langoustine Oil adds a marvellous flavour boost, it goes a long way. A small amount can be substituted for two or three times the amount of fatty mayonnaise or oil dressing used in most seafood dishes.

Langoustine Oil can be used:

- as a replacement for olive oil for dressing pasta
- for finishing a shellfish salad
- for finishing a shellfish risotto
- drizzled over grilled (broiled) lobster (absolutely wonderful!)
- tossed lightly with seafood ravioli
- for a party dip – simply blend 3 tablespoons of Langoustine Oil with 1 tablespoon of balsamic vinegar and use as a dip for every 12 large prawns (shrimp).

This oil must be refrigerated and will keep for no longer than one or two weeks. If you cannot find langoustine, use lobster or crab shells.

MAKES APPROXIMATELY 600 ML (1 PINT/2½ CUPS)

600 ml (1 pint/2½ cups) grapeseed or other high-quality, neutral-tasting oil
*50 g (2 oz/¼ cup) mixed chopped vegetables***
1 sprig each of fresh thyme, flat-leaf parsley (Italian parsley) and lemongrass
1 tsp crushed coriander seeds
1 tsp crushed fennel seeds
2 star anise
*900 g (2 lbs) raw langoustine, lobster or crab shells**
1 tbsp tomato purée (paste)

splash of cognac
900 ml (1½ pints/1 generous quart) water
1 tsp sea salt

1. Place a little of the oil in a pan and lightly fry the mixed vegetables until transparent.
2. Add the herbs, coriander and fennel seeds and star anise and mix.
3. Add the shells and fry for 3–4 minutes, until the shells have changed colour.
4. Add the tomato purée (paste) and stir in.
5. Add the cognac to the pan and light it with a match. Flame until the alcohol has burned off.
6. Remove the pan from the heat.
7. This is the good part! Smash or crush the shells into pieces about the size of your thumbnail. This can be done in a blender or with a wooden mallet. If you use a blender, pulse for no more than 2 minutes. Don't make the pieces too small or the final flavour will taste more of the shells than what they once contained.
8. Slowly incorporate the remaining grapeseed oil and pour into a large saucepan or soup kettle.
9. Add the water and sea salt, place over a high heat and bring to the boil. Boil rapidly for 30 minutes, then remove from the heat.
10. Allow the mixture to cool before pouring it through a strainer, lined with muslin (cheesecloth), into a tall pot or pan. Then, refrigerate for at least 3 hours. The water and oil will separate while the mixture stands.
11. After 3 hours, use a ladle or spoon to lift off the oil. Water will ruin your final product, so it is better to leave a little oil behind than accidentally damage the infusion.
12. Pass the oil you have lifted from the mixture through a fine strainer and then pour it into a sterilized bottle with a tight-fitting cap.

** Use raw shells because they impart a deeper flavour. You can also use small live green crabs or lobster shells.*
*** For the right flavour, use what the French call mirepoix, which includes a small amount of leek, shallot, carrot, fennel and garlic.*

Vinaigrettes

The pleasures of eating fresh vegetables or meat salads or fish can be heightened by dressing them with a well-balanced vinaigrette. These cold dressings, based on what is called an emulsion (the temporary combination of an oil and an acidic liquid, such as lemon juice, vinegar or a very young wine) contribute a smooth background texture to these foods, while adding an unmistakable contrast to their taste. And, because salt is always a part of a vinaigrette, the acid and savoury characteristics of the dressing excite the tongue and accentuate the sensation of flavour.

Making a good vinaigrette

Cooking is all about getting the balance right between hard and soft, sweet and sour, moist and crispy and it requires a little imagination. Select your oil and acidic liquid with care. Begin by considering the main foods in the dish you are about to prepare. Then consider the flavour tones and 'weight' of the various oils you have available. Will virgin olive oil overpower the taste of the dish you are preparing? Would a neutral oil be better? For fish, a grapeseed or soya oil may be a good choice as a base for a vinaigrette, whereas for a salad or roast vegetable dish, olive or nut oil might bring out the garden tastes you want to emphasize.

Next, consider the acidic complement to the oil. The juice from citrus fruit may go well with fish, while for roasted peppers (bell peppers) or asparagus a rich, fine-quality balsamic vinegar with olive oil would be very good. Try new combinations – hazelnut oil and sherry vinegar, for example – before using them to dress a plate. Then, consider the final effect. You may find the latter combination to be a good choice for a sliced egg salad, but the sherry may be wrong for a wholemeal (wholewheat) pasta salad, for which nut oil combined with fresh orange juice may be a better choice.

Vinaigrettes are easy to make, but the following tips will help you maximize their taste.

- Dissolve the salt and any sugar you include in the acidic liquid ingredient of the vinaigrette first, then add the herbs or other flavourings – such as mustard – and finally add the oil.

- Most vinaigrettes are an emulsion of oil and water. By placing the ingredients directly into a screw-top jar, the mixture can be shaken vigorously to mix them thoroughly to achieve the desired effect.
- Vinaigrette does not last long, even with good refrigeration. Make only what you plan to use over a period of one or two days. However, if you love salads, you will probably find that a good vinaigrette gets used very quickly.

There are two sorts of vinaigrette: unemulsified and emulsified. Simple mixtures of oil and vinegar are unemulsified and no matter how hard and long you shake them, they separate into watery and oily layers if left to stand. If an ingredient is added that helps bind the two – mustard and egg yolk are examples – you can achieve a smooth-looking mixture for longer. You will find recipes for both types here. Remember, if a recipe calls for egg yolk, make only what you need for that day. Also, I suggest using pasteurized egg yolks if you are worried about using raw eggs, but, even then, chill the vinaigrette and use it within four to five hours.

Tomato Vinaigrette

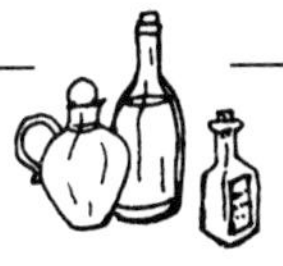

This versatile condiment amplifies the best characteristics of olive oil and balsamic vinegar by adding the refreshing flavours of herbs to ripe tomatoes. Try it as a dressing on simple salads or grilled (broiled) fish.

This vinaigrette will keep for two days in the refrigerator.

MAKES 300 ML (10 FL OZ/1¼ CUPS)

*6 large, very ripe Roma (plum) tomatoes**
1 tbsp chopped fresh coriander or basil
1 tbsp balsamic vinegar (at least 2 years old)
6 tbsp extra virgin olive oil
1 tsp sea salt (or more or less to taste)
freshy ground black pepper

1. Skin the tomatoes by plunging a fork into them, lowering them into boiling water for 15 seconds, then removing them and plunging them straight into a bowl of ice water. The skins will then peel off with ease.
2. Cut the tomatoes in half and squeeze out the seeds.
3. Coarsely chop the fleshy part of the tomatoes and place in a bowl containing all the other ingredients. Using a potato masher, mash them all together well.**

** I prefer using Roma (plum) tomatoes because of their deep flavour and meaty consistency. However, if none are on hand, very ripe beefsteak tomatoes will do.*
*** Although the vinaigrette can be made in a blender, I prefer the chunky consistency produced by using a potato masher.*

Chinese-style Vinaigrette

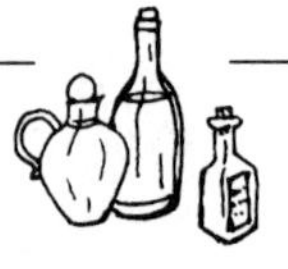

This vinaigrette is one of my favourites. It is excellent with deep-fried Vegetable Beignets (see page 44). Also try it with Chinese-style Monkfish Ravioli (see page 83) or Duck Confit (see page 88). For a quick flavour pick-me-up, sprinkle it over lightly fried squid, grilled (broiled) white fish or toss with rice, some toasted almonds and a few snips of chive or spring onion (scallion). I am sure you will find it to be a handy addition to your bag of cookery tricks!

MAKES 300 ML (10 FL OZ/1¼ CUPS)

2 tablespoons flower honey
juice of 4 limes
1 teaspoon finely chopped garlic
1 tablespoon finely chopped fresh root ginger
1 tablespoon finely chopped fresh horseradish
1 teaspoon soy sauce
*1 teaspoon fish sauce**
4 tablespoons roasted sesame oil
4 tablespoons grapeseed or other neutral oil
small amounts of chopped fresh coriander, finely chopped spring onions (scallions) and sesame or poppy seeds

1. Place the honey in a small saucepan and bring to the boil. Caramelize it slowly. This will take 3–4 minutes, and you want to take it off the heat when the honey has turned a golden colour.

2. Add the lime juice and garlic.

3. Place the ginger and horseradish in another small saucepan, cover with water and bring to the boil. Boil for 1 minute. Blanching them tones down the flavour somewhat, which would otherwise be overpowering.

4. Strain the ginger and horseradish mixture and rinse with cold water.

5. Combine the honey, lime and garlic mixture with the ginger and horseradish.

6. Add the soy sauce and fish sauce.
7. Using a whisk, blend in the sesame and grapeseed, or other, oils.
8. To finish this vinaigrette, add the coriander, spring onions (scallions) and sesame or poppy seeds a few minutes before serving – add them as late as possible so they keep their fresh colour and taste.

** Fish sauce is an oriental ingredient particularly popular in Thailand and is made with anchovies, salt and water. It is a good alternative to salt when you do not really want to use standard seasoning or soy sauce.*

Sharp Red Wine and Walnut Oil Vinaigrette

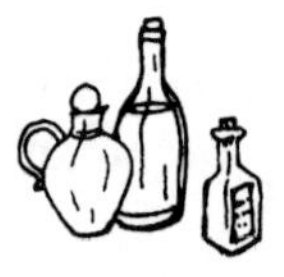

This very light dressing is delicious with duck, smoked chicken breast and wild salmon. Also, try it on:

- a salad of fresh green beans, asparagus and walnuts
- grilled (broiled) goats' cheese with spinach salad
- monkfish.

MAKES 175 ML (6 FL OZ/¾ CUP)

1 tbsp very finely diced shallots
*8 tbsp full-bodied red wine**
*about 1 tsp sugar***
4 tbsp good-quality walnut oil
sea salt and freshly ground black pepper

1. Cook the finely diced shallots over a low heat in a little vegetable oil for 3–5 minutes, or until transparent.
2. Add the red wine and cook over a medium heat until almost all of the fluid has been absorbed by the shallots – there should be about 1 tablespoon of reduction left in the pan.
3. Remove from the heat and add the sugar.
4. Whisk in the walnut oil.
5. Season with salt and pepper. Simple!

** This is a good way to use up the last of a bottle of red wine – it will still be all right even if it has stood, uncorked, all night!*
*** Sugar is often used to cut the acidity of other ingredients, such as wine and tomatoes.*

Aioli with Saffron

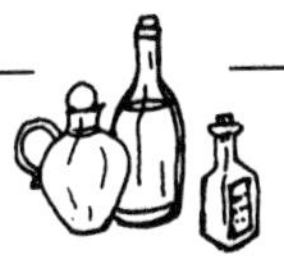

Aioli is garlic-flavoured mayonnaise and it can be used as a dip or as a finish for vegetable stew, which is a traditional dish of the South of France. If you want to try using it as a finish for a stew, add it just before serving, off the heat (or it will curdle), and it will thicken the liquid nicely and add flavour. Aioli with Saffron also goes well with monkfish.

Aioli can be prepared in a blender, a food processor or by hand with a pestle and mortar. The latter is the old-fashioned, but, in my estimation, the best way because you can watch as the ingredients combine and judge the developing texture of the mayonnaise.

MAKES 625 ML (21 FL OZ/SCANT 1¼ US PINTS)

6 garlic cloves, peeled
600 ml (1 pint/2½ cups) extra virgin olive oil
large pinch of saffron strands
2 tbsp white wine
3 golf ball-size new potatoes
*4 free-range egg yolks**
1 tsp Dijon mustard
juice of ½ a lemon
sea salt and cayenne pepper
squeeze of lemon juice

1. Infuse the garlic and olive oil over a very low heat for 30 minutes, or until the garlic is soft. Allow to cool for 30 minutes.
2. At the same time, in a warm place or over a low heat, infuse the saffron in the white wine for 5–10 minutes.
3. Boil and peel the new potatoes. Make sure they are well cooked.
4. Place the fresh egg yolks, mustard, softened garlic and potatoes in a mortar and, with the pestle, work to a smooth paste. This will take about 5 minutes.**

5. Slowly add the saffron in its wine, then slowly drizzle in the cooled oil used to soften the garlic, working it in with the pestle the whole time. If the mixture becomes too thick, add a little warm water.
6. When all of the oil has been incorporated, season with salt and a pinch of cayenne pepper and add a squeeze of fresh lemon juice.

** Pasteurized egg yolk can be substituted if you are worried about using fresh eggs, but the final product will not be as fine. Simply follow the directions on the package regarding what quantity to use.*
*** If you are in a hurry and don't mind missing the pleasure of seeing your mayonnaise emerge before your eyes, use a blender instead. Place all of the ingredients – except the oil – in a blender, give them a quick turn to mix them together well, then slowly add the oil. Adjust the thickness with water if necessary.*

Walnut Oil Dressing

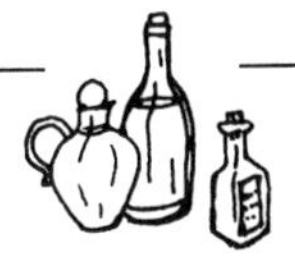

This delicious combination of tastes is ideal for dressing green beans, a salad of fresh peas and broad (fava) beans or dishes made with quail, rabbit or duck. Try Walnut Oil Dressing as a vegetable dip and as a sauce for steamed asparagus. For healthy eating, remember that good walnut oil is an excellent source of essential fatty acids.

When stored in a screw-top bottle or jar or a bowl covered with clingfilm (plastic wrap), this dressing will keep in the refrigerator for two to three days.

MAKES 375 ML (13 FL OZ/SCANT ¾ US PINT)

2 free-range egg yolks (see page 22)
½ teaspoon Dijon mustard
*splash sherry vinegar**
150 ml (5 fl oz/generous ½ cup) walnut oil
150 ml (5 fl oz/generous ½ cup) grapeseed oil
1 tsp hot water
sea salt and freshly ground black pepper

1. Place the egg yolks, mustard and sherry vinegar in a bowl. Whisk them together vigorously.
2. Still whisking, slowly add the walnut and grapeseed oils. Finish** with the hot water.
3. Season to taste with salt and pepper.

** I find that only good-quality sherry vinegar adequately balances the rich flavour of the walnut oil.*
*** The addition of a small amount of hot water here gives a better end product because it slightly dilutes the mixture and adds to the emulsion formed by the egg and oils.*

Green Peppercorn Nappage

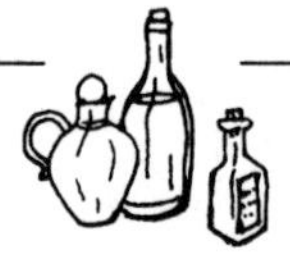

Simple flavour combinations are often the best. This easy dressing combines the taste of two citrus fruits for maximum 'punch'.

Use this *nappage* as a sauce or dressing for salmon, or to marinate fish or chicken. Try brushing it over prawns (shrimp) before grilling (broiling), delicious!

MAKES 135 ML (4½ FL OZ/GENEROUS ½ CUP)

juice of 1 lime
½ tsp soft green peppercorns (sold in jars in brine), drained and crushed with the blade of a knife
60 ml (2 fl oz/¼ cup) extra virgin olive oil
*60 ml (2 fl oz/¼ cup) Colonna granverde**

1. Place all the ingredients in a screw-top bottle and shake well. That's it!

** This is an Italian olive oil that has been pressed together with non-treated lemons, giving it a unique aroma and flavour. Expensive? Yes, but excellent on raw or grilled (broiled) fish and salads. If it is not available near you, infuse extra virgin olive oil with the zest from 2 untreated lemons in a warm place for 4–5 hours before making this recipe.*

Essential ingredients

Making the change from cooking with butter and cream to oils is simplified by keeping a few basic ingredients on hand. These fill the mouth with flavour and the satisfying sensation of oil they leave on the tongue makes the absence of butter or other forms of saturated fat undetectable. Although each ingredient is prepared with oil, they are relatively low in fat and, because a little goes a long way, add few calories to the main dish.

Keep a supply of Tomato Petals, Roasted Garlic and Cherry Tomato Confit in your refrigerator and you will find a dozen ways to use them every week. Tomato Petals, for example, lift the colour and nutritional value of a simple salad, while Roasted Garlic – warmed, crushed with a fork and spread over warm bread – makes a fine accompaniment for a meal of pasta and red wine.

The recipes for these essential ingredients take a bit of time because they require slow cooking in a warm oven, but with a little planning, this can be fitted around ordinary meal preparation. Prepare a casserole, for example, and leave the oven on low while you eat to prepare the garlic, and, perhaps, a tray of Tomato Petals.

Tomato Petals

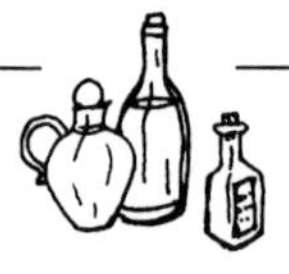

Many of the recipes in this book call for dried tomatoes. You can buy sun-dried tomatoes, but they tend to be too hard for most dishes. Some I have tried are almost inedible. Even softening them in water does not give you an ideal product. We make our own tomato confit, or Tomato Petals, because drying the flesh of the fruit in the oven intensifies its natural flavour and produces a pleasant texture that contrasts nicely with other ingredients.

It is difficult to give specific amounts for the ingredients because this is the kind of recipe that can be tailored to the cooking time you have available and the quantity of tomatoes you have on hand. For example, I like to place my tray of Tomato Petals at the bottom of a low oven while other food is cooking and find that this is a great way to preserve a summer harvest of home-grown tomatoes. So, do as few or as many as you like. If you have time, though, I suggest making as many as possible. Just store them away in the refrigerator and you will find that they will be used up fast enough.

For a delicious snack, spread slices of French bread with Black Olive Tapenade (see page 40), top with Tomato Petals and place under a hot grill (broiler) until the edges of the bread are brown.

Stored in a refrigerator, Tomato Petals will keep for two to three weeks. To avoid deterioration, always make sure the oil covers the Tomato Petals completely.

MAKES 24

6 ripe, firm Roma (plum) tomatoes
good sea salt
a few sprigs of fresh thyme
1 garlic clove, sliced thinly crosswise
3 tbsp extra virgin olive oil

1. Preheat the oven to 110°C/225° F/gas ¼.

2. The tomatoes need to be ripe, and by ripe I mean very red – but not soft. That is imperative. Blanch them in boiling water for 15 seconds, then plunge into ice water and remove the skins.

3. Cut each tomato vertically into quarters. Cut out the seeds and central core (see page 59 for a recipe that uses these). The crescents of tomato flesh are the petals.
4. Place the petals on a baking sheet lined with either foil or baking parchment and sprinkle with sea salt.
5. Break up the fresh thyme and sprinkle it and the thin slices of garlic over the petals.
6. Drizzle with the extra virgin olive oil and place in the preheated oven for 2–3 hours, or until they are nicely shrivelled. What you are doing here is drawing out all of the water and leaving behind the character and body of the tomato.
7. When the petals are dry, remove them from the baking sheet and place in an airtight container or sterilized jar and cover with olive oil.

Roasted Garlic

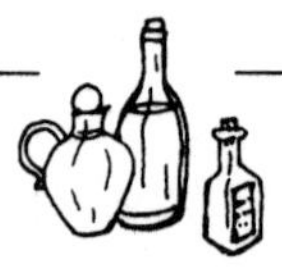

This simple recipe produces a highly versatile and delicious condiment that complements a wide variety of foods – from baked aubergine (eggplant) to freshly baked bread and grilled (broiled) fish. As medical evidence suggests garlic is good for the heart, this is an easy way to increase the number of ways you and your family can enjoy this distinctive ingredient.

A few quick tips for using Roasted Garlic:

- place a few cloves of Roasted Garlic in a blender, add some extra virgin olive oil, whiz for a minute, then add to vegetable soup or ratatouille – the roasted flavour adds a special touch to the final dish
- for an appetizing accompaniment to serve with pasta or salad, sprinkle slices of hot, freshly baked bread with olive oil and spread with crushed Roasted Garlic
- serve with roasted vegetables
- serve with roast chicken and it boosts the flavour.

These delicious 'pearls' keep for several weeks in your refrigerator.

MAKES 18–24

2 heads of garlic
3 tbsp extra virgin olive oil, plus extra as required
sea salt and freshly ground black pepper

1. Preheat the oven to 200°C/400°F/gas 6.
2. Separate the heads of garlic into cloves, but do not peel them. Lay the cloves over the bottom of an ovenproof dish that is just large enough to hold them and drizzle the 3 tablespoons of olive oil over them. Season liberally with salt and pepper.
3. Roast in the preheated oven for 20 minutes, or until the cloves are soft. Remove from the oven and set to one side.

4. Once the cloves have cooled, peel and place them in a clean, dry screw-top container. Pour in more virgin olive oil until they are covered.*

** Olive oil acts as a preservative and, as long as the food is covered with it, protects it from invading bacteria.*

Cherry Tomato Confit

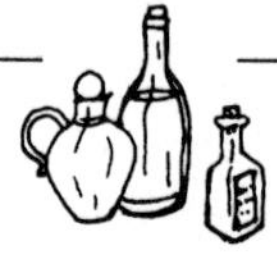

Either red or yellow cherry tomatoes are suitable for this simple garnish. Use only the best tomatoes you can find; those freshly picked from your own garden are ideal. Cherry Tomato Confit can be used:

- hot, as a garnish for lamb or grilled (broiled) chicken breasts
- cold, with a salad.

Warning: these are delicious, so make extra!

These tomatoes will keep very well in the refrigerator for one or two days.

MAKES 15–20

2 tbsp extra virgin olive oil
1 tbsp Pistou (see page 38)
225 g (8 oz) whole cherry tomatoes
salt and freshly ground black pepper

1. Preheat the oven to 200°C/400°F/gas 6.
2. Brush the inside of an ovenproof dish with some of the olive oil and some of the Pistou.
3. Place the cherry tomatoes in the bottom of the dish and brush with the remaining Pistou.
4. Season with salt and pepper and drizzle the remaining virgin olive oil over the tomatoes.
5. Place in the preheated oven and bake for 20–30 minutes, or until the tomatoes have started to shrivel and are completely cooked.

Sauces and savoury toppings

Sauces and savoury toppings made with oils are useful additions to any larder. I have chosen three of the most versatile for inclusion in this collection of recipes: Pistou, the sauce with a thousand uses; Black Olive Tapenade, simple to make and a blessing for cooks in a hurry; and Mushroom Tapenade, a simple cooking ingredient especially created for this collection.

Learn to make these simple recipes and you will be well on your way to creating lighter, healthier food. In Chapter 3, they are used in a variety of surprising ways: the Pistou finds its way into soup and vegetable dishes and the Mushroom Tapenade is served with chicken. I give some suggestions here as to how they can be used to get you started, but experiment in your own kitchen and you will be surprised just how useful they are.

When you use these toppings, you need add no other fat, other than perhaps a little light oil for texture. Saturates are offstage in this show!

Pistou

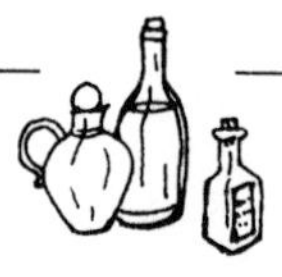

Pistou is a versatile and traditional condiment from Provence, which should not be confused with its close Italian cousin, pesto. The French variety blends the simple flavours of oil, herbs and garlic, while the latter includes Parmesan cheese, which may be too pungent for many dishes. The names of both sauces are derived from the Italian word *pestare,* which means to pound.

This easy-to-make sauce is a key ingredient in many of the recipes that follow, but you will soon find your own ways to incorporate it into your everyday cooking. Try tossing Pistou into freshly cooked pasta and sprinkling toasted pine nuts over or spread it on thick slices of French bread, sprinkle with olive oil and place under the grill (broiler) for a minute. Both are delicious.

The Pistou will keep well in the refrigerator for two to three weeks.

MAKES 175 ML (6 FL OZ/¾ CUP)

2 bunches of basil
*150 ml (5 fl oz/generous ½ cup) extra virgin olive oil**
2 large garlic cloves

1. Pull the basil leaves from the stems, wash them, then plunge into boiling salted water for 15 seconds. Lift the leaves from the water and plunge into ice water. Remove the leaves and squeeze out the excess water.**
2. Pour the oil into a blender.
3. Prepare the garlic by first peeling the cloves, then, with the tip of a knife, removing the germ from the centre of each clove.*** Slice the garlic and place in the blender with the oil.
4. Blend the oil and garlic at high speed for 1 minute, then add the basil and mix for a further minute. The final product can be as fine or as coarse as you like.
5. Spoon the Pistou into a clean, screw-top jar and store in the refrigerator.

* *Your choice of oil will greatly influence the flavour of the Pistou. Use high-quality virgin oil for the best results.*

*** Basil is a 'soft' herb and its leaves discolour when bruised. This procedure preserves the deep green of fresh basil and makes a better-looking final product. Moving the leaves from one stage to the next can be a bit fiddly, unless you first loosely 'package' them in a piece of muslin (cheesecloth) or a nylon strainer.*

**** The garlic 'germ' is that small, elongated bit of green located in the centre of the clove, near the base, which you see when you slice the clove. This is the 'embryo' of the next generation of garlic and so contains many of the substances that give the plant its distinctive, pungent flavour and smell. When garlic cloves age, the germ darkens in colour and grows in size and the garlicky characteristics intensify. If the clove is sliced sideways and the germ removed, the remaining white portion provides a pure garlic flavour without an excessive amount of 'pong'. Also, some people find garlic easier to digest when the germ has been removed.*

Black Olive Tapenade

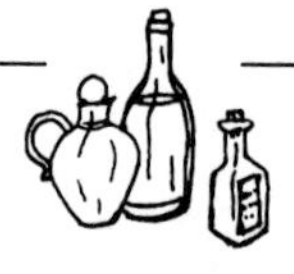

A luscious black with a wonderful savoury taste, this excellent tapenade is such a useful basic ingredient to keep in your refrigerator. In addition to its uses in the recipes in this book, try spreading it on warm bread as an after-school or after-work snack or use it as a sauce for fresh pasta – just sprinkle with some shavings of Parmesan and serve!

This tapenade can be made either in a pestle and mortar, with a knife or in a blender processor, depending on how fine you like it. I prefer to make it with a knife, but see which method suits you best.

Cover the surface of the finished tapenade with olive oil and it will keep for several weeks in the refrigerator.

MAKES APPROXIMATELY 350 ML (12 FL OZ/1½ CUPS)

1 garlic clove
2 anchovy fillets, washed and dried
100 g (4 oz) black olives (stoned/pitted)
1 tsp capers
1 tsp French mustard (Dijon is best)
6 tbsp extra virgin olive oil

1. Crush the garlic clove with the anchovies to form a thick paste.
2. Mix the olives and capers together and chop into fine pieces.
3. Blend these two mixtures together in a mortar, small bowl or blender.
4. Add the French mustard and stir in the extra virgin olive oil. Spoon into a clean screw-topped jar and refrigerate.

Mushroom Tapenade

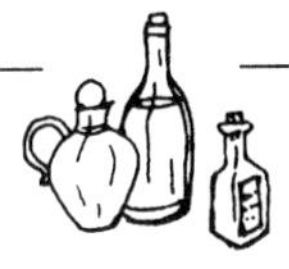

Created for this recipe collection, Mushroom Tapenade is delicious when stirred into pasta or warmed as a dip or thinned with some Mushroom Oil (see page 17) and spread on hot bread. It also makes a fine omelette filling, is appetizing spread on freshly baked bread that has been sliced and brushed with Mushroom Oil, and serves as a fine accompaniment for grilled (broiled) fish, chicken and roasted vegetables.

Omit the anchovies if you wish. Vegetarians and vegans will find this recipe useful because its earthy flavour blends well with grains and pulses (legumes).

Covered with non-PVC clingfilm (plastic wrap) or a container lid, this tapenade can be kept in the refrigerator for three to four days; covered with a little Mushroom Oil, it will keep for one to two weeks.

MAKES 800 G (1¾ LBS)

1 tbsp virgin olive oil (one with a good, strong flavour)
600 g (1½ lbs) button or brown cap mushrooms (wild are best)
1 tbsp chopped shallots
1 garlic clove, finely chopped
2 tbsp capers
1 tbsp Dijon mustard
6 anchovy fillets, washed and dried
8 tbsp Mushroom Oil (see page 17)
1 tbsp fresh chervil
1 tbsp fresh tarragon
sea salt and freshly ground black pepper

1. Heat the virgin olive oil in a frying pan and add the mushrooms. Cook over a high heat until they appear dry. This will take a few minutes, because mushrooms contain a considerable amount of water.

2. When the mushrooms are dry, add the chopped shallots and season to taste with salt and pepper. Add the chopped garlic.*

3. Remove the pan from the heat and place the mushrooms in a blender** with the capers, mustard and anchovies. Blend at a slow speed while adding the Mushroom Oil.
4. Remove the mixture from the blender and finish by mixing in the chopped herbs. If necessary, adjust the seasoning.

** Balance the salt and pepper before adding the garlic or it will be hard to assess the taste accurately.*
*** Strong hands and arms can replace the blender if you want a tapenade with a more chunky, rustic look.*

The final few

There are four further fundamental recipes that I think you will find useful in order to make the most of cooking with oils. The first is a very simple batter for deep frying. When it is done properly and the cooked foods are drained well, deep frying in a light batter can turn simple pieces of fruit, vegetables or fish into mouthwatering treats to enjoy before or during a meal. Just remember, food tastes best when cooking oils are fresh.

The recipe for Fennel Stock is a great base for sauces, soups and stews. Fennel adds a fresh undertone to the taste of foods and this easy recipe greatly increases your flexibility in using and enjoying its benefits. Making your own stock sounds like a lot of work, but in fact it is simple to make and takes little thought once you have learned the basic method. Cubes and granules are easy, but they cannot give the same quality of flavour to a dish.

Two other recipes are Basic Pasta and Basic Polenta. You can buy good freshly made pasta today, but making your own is worth the effort – it has special pizzazz. It is also a great way to introduce children to cooking. With a quick sauce – Pistou, for example – they can put together a gourmet meal from scratch and really impress their friends. The earlier you get kids cooking the better!

It was difficult to decide which grains to include in this collection of fundamental recipes. Risotto is a favourite, as are tabboulé and couscous. However, I finally decided on polenta because it lends itself to more unusual dishes – the Polenta Tart with Tomatoes and Sardines (see page 71), for example. Also, from the standpoint of nutrition, polenta has much to offer. Made from beautiful, yellow maize, polenta is loaded with energy, vitamins and minerals.

Rice Batter for Deep Frying

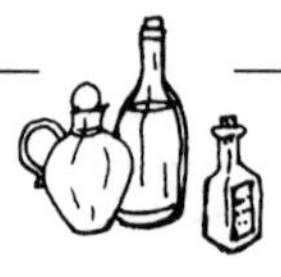

This recipe produces a light, crisp batter with characteristics similar to those of tempura – a light Japanese batter. However, the mustard and herb give a modern flavour that adds some excitement. Unlike other recipes I have tried, this batter does not go soggy.

Use this batter for:

- frying small pieces of squid, sardines, prawns (shrimp) and other seafood, such as Mackerel Beignets (see page 81)
- frying pieces of fruit, such as apple and banana (top with honey)
- Vegetable Beignets (see below).

MAKES 250 ML (8 FL OZ/1 CUP)

125 g (5 oz/1 cup) rice flour
120 ml (4 fl oz/½ cup) ice cold water
1 egg yolk
1 tsp chopped fresh tarragon
1 tbsp tarragon vinegar
2 tsp wholegrain Pommery mustard

1. This is simplicity itself! Place all of the ingredients in a bowl and whisk for about 20 seconds. (You can use a blender, but I enjoy whisking.)

Vegetable Beignets

Try making courgette (zucchini) beignets [do not use the centre of the courgette (zucchini), as it is full of water] or fry baby sweetcorn that has been marinated in soy sauce.

Prepare cauliflower and broccoli in the following way. Steam them for a few minutes, dry them on paper kitchen towel, then dip them in the batter and fry (you want these vegetables to be partially cooked but still crunchy before frying). Cauliflower is my favourite vegetable cooked this way. We marinate it in a small amount of balsamic vinegar and some chopped parsley before dipping it in the batter and deep frying.

All of these vegetables make fine accompaniments for fish, roasted poultry or before-dinner drinks.

Fennel Stock

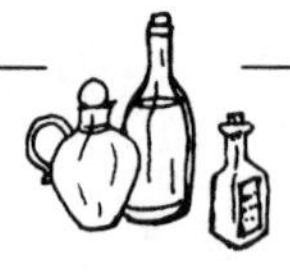

This highly versatile stock can be used as a base for vegetarian soups, vegetarian risotto or sauces to go with fish or chicken.

This stock can be kept in the refrigerator for two to three days or frozen for three to four months.

MAKES 900 ML (24 FL OZ/3 CUPS) STOCK

450 g (1 lb) fennel, chopped
50 g (2 oz/½ cup) shallots, chopped
25 g (1 oz/¼ cup) leek, chopped
2 tbsp extra virgin olive oil
1 sprig of fresh thyme
1 sprig of fresh parsley
1 tsp crushed coriander seeds
1 tsp fennel seeds
2 tsp star anise
pinch of sea salt
2 pieces of lemon zest
900 ml (24 fl oz/3 cups) water

1. In a stock pan, place the vegetables and olive oil and cook over a medium heat until the vegetables are transparent.
2. Add all the other ingredients to the pan and pour in the water.
3. Bring to the boil, then simmer very gently for 20 minutes. Skim and remove the pan from the heat. Allow to cool to room temperature.
4. Strain the stock through a strainer lined with muslin (cheesecloth) or one with a fine mesh. Extract all the goodness from the cooked herbs and vegetables by gently pressing them against the sides of the strainer with the back of a wooden spoon.

Basic Pasta

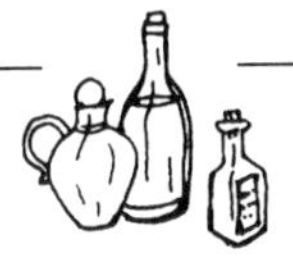

Pasta is an ancient invention, dating back as far as the Chinese Shang Dynasty, 3,500 years ago. Contrary to popular belief, pasta on its own is not fattening – putting too much oil, cream or cheese on top is what will do the damage!

Perhaps the original fast food, cooked pasta can be topped with anything from tomato, garlic and a little olive oil, to a blend of plumped raisins and toasted pine nuts with a drizzle of good-quality olive oil and a generous grating of black pepper and Parmesan cheese. It is truly one of the great foods of the world.

Making pasta is fun, and a great way to introduce children to the pleasures of creating their own food. These days, the equipment needed to prepare noodles is inexpensive and fairly easy to find, so why not experience the real taste of fresh pasta by making your own? This recipe should result in perfect pasta almost every time.

A quick note: fresh pasta should be cooked soon after it is made.

MAKES 300 G (11 OZ)

*250 g (9 oz/scant 2 cups) of durum wheat flour**
2 whole size 3 (large) eggs, plus 2 yolks
a little water
large pinch of salt

1. Place the ingredients in a robo-coup or the bowl of a mixer with a paddle and work into a dough. Alternatively, mix them into a dough in a bowl. You do not want the dough to break when you roll it through the pasta machine, so you are aiming for a dough that is slightly damp; if it looks too dry, add a very small amount of water.

2. When the dough is well blended, form it into a ball, wrap it in clingfilm (plastic wrap) and leave it to rest in the refrigerator for 1 hour to 1 hour 30 minutes.**

3. Roll out the dough. Begin by flattening the rested dough to a thickness of about 1 cm (½ in), then begin rolling it through the pasta machine.*** Going down through the gears of the machine, continue passing the dough through the machine until you have reached the last one.

4. When you have passed the dough through the finest gear, cut it to the size and shape you want and allow it to air-dry. Use as soon as possible, but otherwise store in an air-tight container.

** Durum wheat is ideal for pasta and can be obtained from speciality food stores and most Italian delicatessens (Italian grocers). Make sure to buy the fine-milled OO grade as it is specially ground for pasta.*
*** Resting the dough this way allows it to relax and for all the liquid to be absorbed into the flour. This makes it easier to roll. You may be surprised to find that the dough feels quite firm when it goes into the refrigerator and much softer when you take it out later.*
**** A little tip for rolling out the pasta. When you pass the dough through the machine, you want to avoid using any additional flour. Flour has a tendency to stick to the pasta and not come off and so during cooking it leaves a starchy film which makes the pasta unattractive. At One Paston Place, we use some finely ground semolina when we roll the dough. This not only stops the dough sticking, it allows you to make the pasta dough a little more moist because the semolina absorbs the excess moisture and helps dry it out.*

Herb Pasta

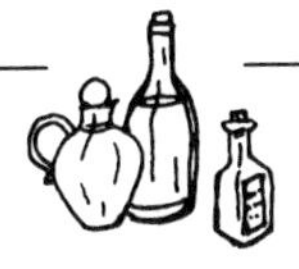

While you are making pasta, try preparing some of this very special variety for Grilled (Broiled) Vegetable Lasagne (see page 63).

MAKES 300 G (11 OZ)

1 quantity Basic Pasta
6 leaves of each of the following: fresh basil, parsley, chervil, coriander, tarragon or other fresh herbs

1. Prepare the Basic Pasta as given above up to step 4.
2. When you have passed the dough through the finest gear, lay out two equal-sized sheets. Over one sheet, liberally scatter the leaves of your choice of herbs (use only the leaves – stems make lumps).
3. Place the second sheet of pasta on top of the scattered herbs and carefully roll this 'herb sandwich' through the *second* finest gear on your machine. Then run the dough through the machine's finest gear. This will impregnate the lasagne with the fresh herbs and give a totally new taste to the sheets of pasta. Cut the sheets into 10 by 5-cm (4 by 2-in) rectangles and dry for later use.

Basic Polenta

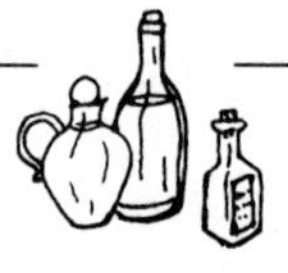

Polenta is finely ground cornmeal and so is rich in vitamins and minerals. There are two types. One involves stirring constantly over a low heat for about an hour, while the other takes about five minutes to cook. I recommend using the quick-cooking variety as I think there is little to be gained from the more laborious process.

500 ml (17 fl oz/1 generous US pint) water with a pinch of sea salt or chicken stock or Fennel Stock (see page 46)
125 g (5 oz) instant polenta
2 tbsp Mushroom Oil (see page 17)
50 g (2 oz) Parmesan cheese, finely grated

1. Bring the water or stock to the boil and sprinkle in the polenta, slowly, stirring. In France they call this process *pluie*, meaning rain, which well describes this simple technique. Stir continuously over a medium heat for 4 minutes.
2. When cooked, stir in the Mushroom Oil and the cheese, then leave to stand for 5 minutes.
3. Turn the polenta out onto a tray that has been well coated with olive oil. As most of the recipes later in this book call for circles of polenta, you can pour the freshly cooked meal onto the tray in 4 equal portions, allow it to cool slightly, then level it off with a pallet knife. Trim the edges if necessary.

VARIATION

Polenta can also be served soft, with a similar consistency to that of mashed potatoes. For this you will need about 750 ml (1¼ pints/generous 1½ US pints) water or stock. Proceed as far as step 2 of the method for Basic Polenta, then serve.

Recipes for Healthy Eating

If you have followed the recipes of the previous two chapters, you now know something about cooking with oils. Perhaps your refrigerator is well stocked with Tomato Petals and Mushroom Oil. For some truly delicious and healthy meals, next turn your hand to the following recipes. Glancing through this chapter you will find that most dishes are built around fresh vegetables and healthy grains and there is no butter in sight – only the fine oils and oil-based foundation recipes described earlier.

Although this collection of recipes was not designed specifically for vegetarians, many of them are ideal for people who want to eliminate meat from their diet. I can particularly recommend the Polenta with Grilled (Broiled) Asparagus and Wild Mushrooms, the Grilled (Broiled) Vegetable Lasagne and the Spring Vegetable Soup.

For those meat eaters among you, there are ways to cook quail, chicken, duck and rabbit. I like quail and rabbit; they both have good lean meat. As for duck, the fact is that duck fat is rather similar to olive oil: it contains twice as much monunsaturated fat as saturated fat and, surprisingly, contains polyunsaturated fat as well, so is not as bad for you as you may previously have thought.

There are several recipes for fish, most of which use the oily varieties as we should all eat oily fish at least once a week. Many people avoid eating these fish because they find them dull or too 'fishy'. If you are one of these, look at the recipes for Mackerel Beignets and Fresh Tuna Carpaccio (see pages 81 and 74) and see if they could help change your mind. Oily fish can really be very good indeed!

A word about portion sizes

Unless otherwise stated, these recipes make four starter-size portions. This is because I find that many people are looking for smaller portions these days and many recipes make too much to eat comfortably, especially when there are two or more courses. Most of these recipes, though (except the Marinated Side of Salmon and Hot-smoked Fillet of Wild Salmon), can be doubled up if you wish to serve bigger portions.

Snacks, soups and easy starters

Most snacks and starters have two things in common: we usually eat them when we are hungry and our appetites are at their peak; and they can be loaded with unseen saturated fats. Follow the next three recipes and you will have some nutritious light treats that the entire family will enjoy.

Deep-fried Root Vegetables

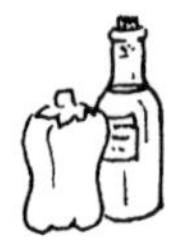

This is one of my all-time favourite recipes. Easy to make and delicious, these vegetable crisps (chips) are nutritious into the bargain! Making and munching your way through a stack of them is an ideal way to pass some good family time.

They work well as a snack, as an attractive topping for salads, as a pre-dinner starter with drinks and as high-energy food for hungry children after school. Some of the dip recipes included in this book are excellent when served with them.

SERVES 4–6 PEOPLE

225 g (8 oz) parsnips, peeled
225 g (8 oz) raw beetroot (beet), peeled
225 g (8 oz) sweet potato, peeled
225 g (8 oz) Jerusalem artichokes, peeled
225 g (8 oz) carrots, peeled
225 g (8 oz) celeriac (celery root), peeled
sea salt

You can also include:

225 g (8 oz) white potatoes, peeled*
*225 g (8 oz) globe artichokes***

1. Peel the vegetables and slice them very thinly using either a mandoline*** or other slicing machine. Slicing them by hand results in the slices being of varying thicknesses and so does not give a good finished product. You can slice the vegetables either widthways, making round, more or less circular shapes, or lengthwise, creating rather longer shapes. The shape does not matter, but what is important is that the slices from all of the vegetables are the same thickness as much as possible so they cook evenly.

2. Prepare your fryer – this can be a self-contained electric fryer or a heavy-based saucepan with about 1.5 litres (2½ pints/3 US pints and ¼ cup) vegetable oil in it – and heat until it reaches 150–170°C/300–325°F). Remember, never fill a saucepan more than one third full with oil.

3. Cook the vegetables, deep frying each variety separately, one at a time. Several of these vegetables have a high water content and so need to be cooked twice – remember, the best crisps (potato chips) in the world are always fried twice because they crisp up better and stay crisper longer.
   Also, these vegetables have different cooking times. Plan to cook the beetroot (beet), celeriac (celery root) and Jerusalem artichokes twice (these all have a high water content). The parsnip, sweet potato and carrot slices will need to be fried only once. With the exception of the beetroot (beet), I suggest beginning with the vegetables that need frying twice. The beetroot (beet) discolours the oil so if you fry it first, it will colour the other crisps (chips). I suggest you begin by frying the slices of Jerusalem artichoke, then the celeriac (celery root).
   Depending on the type of fryer you use, place the appropriate amount of slices into the frying basket and be ready to lower them into the hot oil. When the oil has reached between 150 and 180°C/300 and 350°F, plunge in the slices of Jerusalem artichoke and cook until the oil has stopped bubbling or fizzing, 2–3 minutes. Then, remove the Jerusalem artichoke slices from the oil and spread them out to drain on paper kitchen towel on a tray. When they are dry, return them to the fryer and cook them again. After the second frying, the slices should be completely dry and crisp. Repeat with the celeriac (celery root), then reheat the oil again to 180°C/350°F and cook the other vegetables (I usually cook the parsnips next). As each batch of crisps (chips) is finished, lift them out of the oil very quickly and spread them out to drain on a fresh piece of paper kitchen towel. Continue with all of the vegetables, twice-frying the beetroot (beet) last.
4. When all of the vegetables are crispy and golden brown, sprinkle them lightly with salt and mix together. You will then have a colourful assortment of vegetable crisps (chips) that can be served as they are, as topping on a salad or main course or dipped into any number of delicious sauces. Some good dips are:

- Black Olive Tapenade (see page 40) – simply thin with a little extra virgin olive oil and mix in a little chopped spring onion (scallion) for bite and texture
- Aioli with Saffron (see page 27)
- Chinese-style Vinaigrette (see page 24)
- Walnut Oil Dressing (see page 29).

** I like Maris Piper, but you can use any potato suitable for frying.*

*** These are quite expensive and not easy to cut, but have a wonderful flavour when deep-fried.*
**** If you use a mandoline – which is my recommendation – be careful because the blades are very sharp. Also, slice varieties of vegetables separately and do not mix as different vegetables have different water contents, which affects their cooking time. Another tip: lay the vegetable slices out on paper kitchen towel in a dry place to help evaporate the moisture released by slicing.*

Spring Vegetable Soup

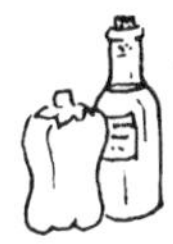

A favourite with both vegetarian and non-vegetarian guests at One Paston Place, this soup combines the earthy flavours of Mushroom Oil with the sweet taste and crisp texture of lightly cooked fresh vegetables.

The quality of the final product depends on the quality of the ingredients you use, so don't skimp – use the best and freshest vegetables you can find.

Freshly baked wholegrain bread is the perfect accompaniment.

SERVES 6

350 ml (12 fl oz/1½ cups) Fennel Stock (see page 46)
225 g (8 oz) wild mushrooms (morels, shiitakes, ceps and some shavings of truffle if the budget allows)
4 tbsp olive oil
*fresh vegetables (vary according to season and location, but try peas, broad (fava) beans, French beans (fine green beans), asparagus and shallots)**
*1 tsp of each of several fresh herbs (coriander, flat-leaf parsley (Italian parsley, chervil and tarragon are good choices)***
*6 fresh artichoke bottoms****
6 tbsp Mushroom Oil (see page 17)
1 tsp truffle oil (optional, but adds marvellous flavour and aroma)
sea salt and freshly ground black pepper

1. Prepare the Fennel Stock according to the recipe on page 46.
2. Sauté the mushrooms in some of the olive oil until all the juices rendered have evaporated.
3. If using, peel and quarter the shallots, place in a pan, cover with cold water and bring to the boil. Cook for 5–6 minutes. Pour into a colander and strain. Pick, shell and blanch the peas and beans, if using, in boiling salted water until tender – 3–4 minutes should do – you do not want them overcooked.
4. Peel the asparagus, if using, and blanch in boiling salted water for 3–5

minutes, depending on the thickness of the stems.

5. Wash the herbs, removing and discarding any stems. Dry and blanch in boiling water for no more than 10 seconds. Drain them in a strainer and rinse the herbs with cold water. Chop them coarsely.
6. Stir-fry the artichoke bottoms in the remaining olive oil.
7. Place the artichoke bottoms and cooked mushrooms in a heavy-based stock pan, add the Fennel Stock and bring to the boil. Cook for 3–5 minutes. Remove from the heat.
8. Add the herbs and the remaining vegetables. Stir in the Mushroom Oil and season with salt and pepper. If you are using truffle oil, add a few drops to each soup plate just before serving.

** You can make this soup fit your dinner plans and your mood. If you want something light to start a meal, keep the quantity of vegetables you use to a minimum – some asparagus and shallots, perhaps. If you want a hearty dish, and feel like trying new flavours, see what is in season and prepare a total of about 175 g (6 oz/generous cup) mixed vegetables per person. Just make certain all the vegetables are lightly cooked before serving. Crispness is essential in this soup.*

*** Although fresh herbs are necessary to achieve the rich balance of aromas and tastes in this soup, use them sparingly so they do not overwhelm the individual tastes of the vegetables.*

**** Artichokes are flower buds. For this dish, we want to use only the soft part of the bud that holds the prickly inner parts of the flower. This takes some skill, but once you have learned the trick of preparing these artichoke bottoms you will find their excellent taste and flavour worth the effort.*

To prepare an artichoke bottom, break off the stem and pull away any tough fibres. Cut off and discard the coarse bottom leaves. Place the artichoke on its side and, working around the artichoke, cut away the side leaves with a sharp knife until the soft, inner flesh is exposed. You only want to remove the leaves; do not remove more than necessary. 'Top' the artichoke by cutting across the upper leaves of the bud. This should leave a round section of artichoke about 2.5 cm (1 in) thick. Trim off all remaining segments of leaves; then scoop out the inner 'choke' – the prickly strands. Rinse. For this dish, place the artichoke bottom on a flat surface and slice it thinly crosswise.

Chilled Tomato Soup

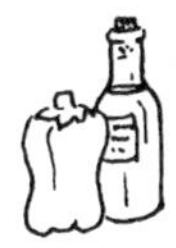

Waste not want not is a saying that holds true in any well-run kitchen. Thus, this recipe shows what you can do with all the cores and seeds that accumulate when you make Tomato Petals (see page 32).

What you have at the end is a lightly flavoured tomato dish that can be served ice-cold as a summer soup or spread around fish or salad as a simple tomato vinaigrette – it can be used for lots of things. Whatever you use it for, it is nice and refreshing, and almost free!

1 kg (2¼ lb) very ripe, Roma (plum) tomatoes, skinned
pinch of sugar, if necessary
2 tsp 8-year-old balsamic vinegar
4 tbsp extra virgin olive oil
sea salt and freshly ground black pepper

1. Put all the tomato trimmings – but not the skins – into a blender. Put on the lid and whiz at high speed for about 2 minutes. Pour the resulting frothy mixture into a fine strainer to remove the remaining seeds. With the back of a wooden spoon, press the mixture gently against the strainer. The result will look like a thick tomato juice. Pour it into a tureen or bowl.

2. Season with salt, pepper, and – if the tomatoes are particularly acidic – a pinch of sugar. Add the balsamic vinegar and extra virgin olive oil. Place in the refrigerator for at least 2 hours or overnight (this improves the flavour and lets the air trapped during blending escape, leaving a richer red colour).

Quick Soupe au Pistou

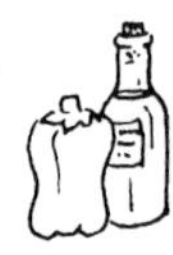

Sprinkled with a little freshly grated Parmesan cheese and served with hot wholemeal (wholewheat) bread, this soup makes a fine meal on a cold winter's day. Busy cooks will appreciate the fact that it tastes even better when made a day ahead or well in advance of being served.

50 g (2 oz/⅓ cup) dried flageolet beans (green haricot beans)
50 g (2 oz/⅓ cup) dried white coco beans (Navy beans)
3 tbsp Pistou (see page 38)
12 Tomato Petals (see page 32)
1 red pepper (bell pepper)
1 yellow pepper (bell pepper)
1 medium aubergine (eggplant)
2 medium courgettes (zucchini)
1 bulb fennel
4–5 tbsp olive oil
½ onion, diced the same size as the rest of the vegetables
900 ml (1½ pints/scant 2 US pints) Fennel Stock (see page 46)
50 g (2 oz/⅓ cup) extra fine green beans, cut into 1-cm (½-in) lengths

1. Soak the flageolet and coco beans in water overnight.
2. Next day, drain the beans, then cook them in fresh slightly salted water for at least 1–1½ hours. If you have a pressure cooker, cook the beans for 15 minutes.
3. Place the Pistou in a mortar. Finely chop the Tomato Petals and crush to a smooth paste.
4. Prepare the vegetables as described in the recipe Provençal Vegetables with Pistou on page 101.
5. In a heavy-based saucepan, heat 2 tablespoons of the olive oil and add the onion, cooked coco and flageolet beans, peppers, aubergine (eggplant) and fennel. Cook over a medium heat, stirring occasionally, until the onion becomes transparent (3–5 minutes).

6. Add the Fennel Stock and bring to the boil. Simmer for 20 minutes.*
7. Add the courgettes (zucchini) and the raw extra fine green beans. Heat for another 5 minutes. Stir in the Pistou and tomato mixture.
8. Ladle into warm soup plates and serve.

> * *If you plan to serve the soup later, or the next day, stop here; reheat to simmering just before serving, and continue as follows.*

Main courses

Among these recipes are many we serve our guests at One Paston Place. I hope you enjoy trying the Hot-smoked Fillet of Wild Salmon and the Duck Confit (see pages 78 and 88).

Some of the recipes look a bit complicated, but do not be alarmed – they are simpler than the length of the instructions imply. Just allow yourself enough time and organize the ingredients before you begin and you will be fine.

A quick note about wild mushrooms

It is best not to have mushrooms sitting around for any length of time, so after you have purchased a quantity for a particular dish, clean and sauté them as described below as soon as you get them home.

Regarding cleaning them, I suggest first inspecting the mushrooms to see if they are free of sand and dirt. If they are pretty clean, brush them lightly with a damp cloth or mushroom brush to remove any debris – and consider yourself lucky. If the mushrooms need cleaning, however, wash them quickly in warm water to remove any mud or sand clinging to them. Mushrooms absorb considerable quantities of water, so the quicker you wash them the better.

As soon as you have cleaned the mushrooms, place them in a pan with a few drops of olive oil and heat them until all of the water has evaporated. Pour into a colander and leave to drain until you are ready to prepare your dish, then sauté them again as required by the recipe.

I do not recommend sautéing mushrooms only once, unless you are using fairly dry varieties, such as oyster or shiitake mushrooms, which are usually cultivated rather than wild and only need a light brushing to clean them.

Grilled (Broiled) Vegetable Lasagne

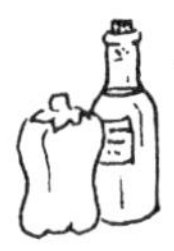

Everyone enjoys this dish, whether they are vegetarian or not. If you leave the egg out of the pasta, then it is perfect for vegans.

You can use sheets of good-quality fresh lasagne, but the Herb Pasta gives an unusual touch.

Which vegetables you include is up to you. I don't think parsnips and carrots would give as good a result, but you could give them a try. Those given in the recipe are those characteristic of the south of France, a place I love so much.

1 red pepper (bell pepper)
1 yellow pepper (bell pepper)
5 tbsp olive oil
1 large aubergine (eggplant)
1 bulb fennel
1 large courgette (zucchini)
2 uncooked artichoke bottoms (see page 58; optional)
8 fresh asparagus spears
8 baby corn cobs
16 sheets of lasagne made from half quantity of fresh Herb Pasta (see page 48)
150 ml (5 fl oz/generous ½ cup) Fennel Stock (see page 46)
some fresh herbs – flat-leaf parsley (Italian parsley), coriander, small amount of tarragon
juice of 1 lemon
4 tbsp Mushroom Oil (see page 17), plus extra to serve
12 Tomato Petals (see page 32)
sea salt and freshly ground black pepper

1. Preheat the oven to 180°C/355°F/gas 4.

2. Begin by roasting the peppers. An easy way to do this is to place the peppers on their sides in a heavy flameproof frying pan, brush them with olive oil and place under a hot grill (broiler) until they blister. Don't worry if they blacken slightly – this adds colour and taste to the final product. Turn the peppers over

and repeat until they are blistered all over. Remove the peppers from the pan and place them in a bowl and cover at once with clingfilm (plastic wrap) or place them in a lidded plastic container. The steam from the hot vegetables will loosen the skins and help lift them away from the flesh. Leave the peppers covered for about 1 hour, then peel them, remove the seeds and cut each into 8 sections.

3. Put a large saucepan with 2 litres (3½ pints/4⅓ US pints), 1 tablespoon of olive oil and 2 teaspoons of sea salt on to boil. Once it is boiling, turn down the heat until the water is very gently simmering, then add half the lasagne sheets and cook them for 3 minutes. Once they have cooked, carefully lift them out and place them in a large bowl full of cold water. Repeat for the remaining lasagne and when they have cooked, drain all the sheets and lay them on a tray or worksurface covered with clingfilm (plastic wrap) and lightly drizzled with a little olive oil to prevent them from sticking. Make sure the sheets are well spaced and cover them with clingfilm (plastic wrap).
4. Cut the aubergine (eggplant), fennel, courgette (zucchini) and – if using – the artichoke bottoms into slices about 3–5 cm/1¼–2 in thick. Place them on a plastic tray or plate and sprinkle a little salt, pepper and olive oil over them.
5. Place the asparagus and baby corn in a separate dish and season in the same way.
6. Grill (broil) the fennel. When cooked, place the fennel, baby corn and asparagus in a shallow baking dish and brush with olive oil. Bake in the preheated oven for 20 minutes, adding the Tomato Petals to the dish for the final 3 minutes of cooking.
7. Meanwhile, lightly brush olive oil over the rack of a charcoal grill, or even a small ridged frying pan, and grill the aubergine (eggplant), courgette (zucchini), peppers and – if using – the artichoke. Make sure they are cooked through.
8. Once cooked, keep the vegetables warm and heat up the sheets of lasagne pasta by either placing them in a steamer or a tray and cover with boiling water. Drain off in a colander. Season the pasta with a little salt and pepper and some olive oil.
9. On 4 plates, build up the lasagne in whatever way you choose. On each plate, lay out a sheet of pasta, top with vegetables; repeat with a second layer, then top with a third sheet of pasta. I usually keep the asparagus, Tomato Petals and baby corn to garnish the lasagne.

10. Next, make a sauce. Pour the Fennel Stock into a saucepan and reduce by one third.
11. Add the herbs to the stock, season with salt, pepper and lemon juice, add the Mushroom Oil and stir together over a medium heat.
12. Remove the sauce from the heat, pour into a blender and blend for 1 minute. The mixture will emulsify and make an attractive, frothy sauce.
13. Cover the lasagne with the warm sauce, float a few drops of Mushroom Oil here and there on the plate and serve. A real crowd pleaser!

Polenta with Grilled (Broiled) Asparagus and Wild Mushrooms

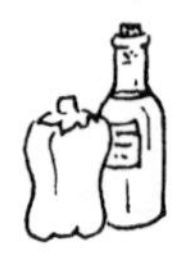

This beautiful dish is a favourite with both vegetarians and non-vegetarians dining at One Paston Place. It is full of flavour and the variety of textures makes this an excellent choice for a dinner party or a special meal with the family.

*900 g (2 lbs) fresh asparagus**
2 tbsp extra virgin olive oil
*225 g (8 oz) wild mushrooms***
approximately 4 tbsp Mushroom Oil (see page 17)
1 tbsp diced shallots
1 tbsp finely chopped chives
4 Basic Polenta circles (see page 50)
a few drops of 8-year-old balsamic vinegar
sea salt and freshly ground black pepper

1. Chargrill the asparagus. Begin by brushing the asparagus with olive oil, sprinkling with salt and pepper and leaving for 1–2 hours. When you are ready, place the asparagus on a hot charcoal grill. Turn every minute or so until the whole stem of the asparagus is lightly browned. The cooking time depends on the size of the asparagus. For spears about the thickness of your little finger, allow about 4 minutes on the grill. Another minute or two in a hot oven will make sure they are cooked through.

2. Sauté the wild mushrooms in 1 tablespoon of the Mushroom Oil and season with salt and pepper. Add the shallots and chives.

3. Heat the Basic Polenta circles by either placing them on a baking sheet in the oven or frying them lightly in a little oil in a non-stick pan.

4. Place a circle of polenta on each of 4 plates and layer your asparagus haphazardly in a criss-crossed manner on top.

5. Divide the mushrooms between the servings, scattering them over the asparagus.

6. Finish each plate by trickling a little Mushroom Oil and a few drops of balsamic vinegar around each circle of polenta.
7. Serve and graciously accept the applause!

** For chargrilling, fine asparagus spears are best as there is no waste.*
*** Most mushroom varieties we think of as 'wild' – oyster and shiitake for example – are, in fact, cultivated. Try to get these if you can. When the shelves are bare, however, mix a few dried wild morels or trompette de la mort with some cultivated field mushrooms. For maximum flavour and texture, choose open-capped mushrooms. See also A quick note about wild mushrooms, page 62.*

Warm Goats' Cheese Salad with Jerusalem Artichoke Crisps (Chips)

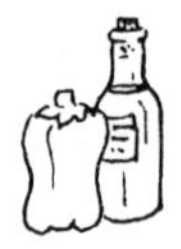

This simple salad is a big favourite in our restaurant. If we take it off the menu, there is always someone who asks for it. Add it to your collection of special dishes, because it is quick, easy, beautiful on the plate and something people truly enjoy.

Unlike a few years ago, there are now many goats' cheeses on the market. The majority are made with vegetarian rennet, so, unless you are a vegan, this is an ideal high-protein meal. It is important, however, to choose a cheese made from full-fat milk because it cooks better. At One Paston Place we use a cheese made locally, in East Sussex, which is very similar to the type of goats' cheese most popular in France. It has a rather firm, white outer crust and becomes very soft at the edges when heated, but remains firm in the centre. The contrasting textures add interest.

1 thin baguette (French bread)
1 or 2 plump garlic cloves
2–3 tbsp olive oil
250-g (9-oz) goats' cheese log
2–3 tbsp Pistou (see page 38)
12 Tomato Petals (see page 32)
a few drops of balsamic vinegar
*185 g (6½ oz) mixed salad leaves, preferably the soft varieties**
25 g (1 oz) soft herbs of your choice (chervil goes particularly well)
1 tbsp pine nuts (sautéd lightly in olive oil)
Jerusalem artichoke crisps (chips) (see page 54), made from 4 large Jerusalem artichokes

1. Prepare the croûtons (they are best when freshly made). Take the thin baguette (French bread) and rub the crust all over with a cut clove of garlic. Continue until the bread is very wet. Day-old bread is ideal for this, as it cuts more easily. Once the bread is saturated with garlic, slice it very thinly, place the slices on a baking sheet, sprinkle with a little olive oil and place under a hot grill (broiler) until browned. Turn over and brown on the other side. Take them out, leave the croûtons on the tray and the grill (broiler) on.

2. Cut the goats' cheese log into 12 equal slices and place 1 on top of each garlic croûton. Make sure the bread is completely covered or it will burn when the croûtons go back under the grill (broiler).
3. Brush the goats' cheese with a little Pistou.
4. Place under the hot grill (broiler) for 2 minutes, or until lightly browned (watch them as they burn easily).
5. Remove the cheese-topped croûtons from under the grill (broiler) and place a Tomato Petal on each.
6. Return to the grill (broiler) for a further 2 minutes. Remove and keep warm.
7. Dress the salad leaves with olive oil and a few drops of balsamic vinegar, then divide between 4 plates, arranging the leaves in a flat fashion so the croûtons will stay where you place them and not tip to the side or fall off the salad.
8. Sprinkle with pine nuts and Jerusalem artichoke crisps (chips).

** Baby spinach is nice with this (make sure the leaves are no bigger than the size of your two thumbs put together), along with a small amount of rocket (arugula), lollo rosso and watercress.*

Fish and seafood

We know there is a direct connection between the fats in our diet and cardiac disease, although the mechanics of this linkage are unclear. While the scientists are busy working out exactly how the chemistry works, we can enjoy eating wonderful fish knowing the oils they contain are the best kind for healthy hearts.

Polenta Tart with Tomato and Sardines

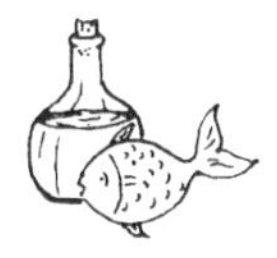

Attractive, economical and packed full of nutritious ingredients, this dish is a hit any time of year.

4 x 10-cm (4-in) Basic Polenta circles (see page 50, made with extra virgin olive oil in place of the Mushroom Oil)
2 tbsp extra virgin olive oil
2 tbsp Black Olive Tapenade (see page 40)
48 Tomato Petals (see page 32)
8 very fresh sardines, each about 10 cm (4 in) long and 100 g (4 oz), filleted
sea salt

1. Preheat the oven to 220°C/425°F/gas 7.
2. To prepare the bases for the tarts, place the Basic Polenta circles on a baking sheet covered with oiled baking parchment (you do not want them to stick, so oil well). Spread the Black Olive Tapenade over the polenta.
3. Arrange 10–12 Tomato Petals on top of each base, overlapping them slightly to form a flower shape.
4. Cut the fish fillets in half to make 8 pieces of fish per tart. Arrange in a flower shape on top of the Tomato Petals.
5. Drizzle some extra virgin olive oil over the fish and sprinkle lightly with sea salt.
6. Place in the preheated oven and bake for 6–8 minutes. The tarts need to be in the oven just long enough to warm them through and cook the sardines. Obviously the size of the sardines will determine the cooking time, but they do cook very quickly.
7. Remove the tarts from the oven and place in the centre of 4 heated plates. Surround with a few drops of extra virgin olive oil or, if you are lucky enough to have some, lemon-flavoured olive oil from Colonna.
8. Serve immediately with a small side salad to complete the meal.

Marinated Side of Salmon

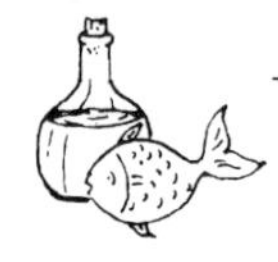

Ideal for Christmas or dinner parties, this is an excellent way to prepare a whole side of salmon. It also works well with tail pieces, although they do not have the same visual appeal.

Use very fresh salmon for this dish and wild salmon if available as the taste and texture of the final product is far better.

This recipe is for one side of salmon, which weighs about 1 kg (2½ lbs) and will feed eight to ten people as a starter at a dinner party. With any luck, you'll have some left over for sandwiches the next day.

This recipe can also be made using seabass (striped bass) or marinated tuna instead of salmon. Pieces weighing between 2 and 2½ kg (4 and 5 lbs) are best. Again, use only the best-quality fish.

50 g (2 oz/generous ¼ cup) sea salt
25 g (1 oz/generous ⅛ cup) caster sugar (granulated sugar)
*1½ tsp badiane (powdered star anise, available in Chinese food shops) or 1 tsp crushed coriander seeds**
juice of ½ a lime
4 tbsp olive oil
*50 g (2 oz) fresh dill or coriander, chopped**
1 side of salmon (about 1 kg/2½ lbs)
freshly ground black pepper
½ quantity Green Peppercorn Nappage (see page 30), to serve
4 tbsp capers, to serve
2 tbsp chopped chives, to serve

1. In a bowl, mix all the chosen ingredients together – except the salmon, pepper, Green Peppercorn *Nappage*, capers and chives. This marinade is thick.

2. Lay the fish on a tray or in a shallow pan, skin-side down. Pat the marinade over the fish, putting the majority over the thickest part of the fillet.

3. Cover the tray with clingfilm (plastic wrap) and place in the refrigerator overnight.

4. The following morning, turn the fish, spoon the marinade over its skin side, return to the refrigerator and leave for a further 8 hours. After this, the fish is ready to serve.

5. Place the fish on a cutting board and scrape off the marinade mixture. With a thin-bladed, sharp knife, cut the fish into very thin slices, working from the head towards the tail.

6. Place the slices on plates, sprinkle liberally with freshly ground black pepper, and brush with the Green Peppercorn *Nappage*. Sprinkle with capers and chopped chives, and serve.

> * *With this recipe, you can produce two quite different dishes. Classically, in Scandinavia, gravad lax is made with dill. When using dill, you also need to use the 1½ teaspoons of badiane. If, on the other hand, you want something more modern and a bit more French, use coriander – omitting the badiane and substituting the 1 teaspoon of crushed coriander seeds. Both are delicious!*

Fresh Tuna Carpaccio

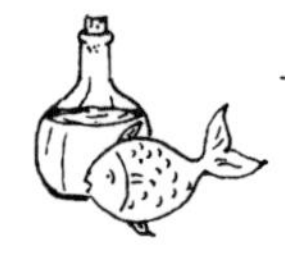

This is an ideal starter for a dinner party. I must stress, though, that freshness is absolutely vital for this dish. You can see if raw tuna is fresh by its colour – it should look much like raw red meat.

350 g (12 oz) fresh tuna
4 tbsp Green Peppercorn Nappage (see page 30)
1 tbsp capers (the smallest you can find)
10 g (¼ oz) fresh horseradish, very finely chopped
2 tbsp chopped chives
sea salt

1. With a very sharp knife or using a slicing machine if you have one, slice the tuna as finely as you can.*
2. Place the tuna slices between 2 sheets of clingfilm (plastic wrap) and pound the slices until they are very thin.**
3. Once the tuna has been flattened, remove the slices from between the sheets of clingfilm (plastic wrap) and divide between 4 large plates. Arrange the slices so that they do not overlap.
4. Gently brush the tuna with the Nappage and scatter the capers over.
5. Cut or shred the fresh horseradish into julienne*** – the finest possible strips – and sprinkle over the fish. Add a sprinkling of chopped chives and a little sea salt to finish.

** Another tip: we place the tuna in the freezer for about an hour, until it becomes very cold, but does not begin to freeze. This gives some solidity to the meat and makes slicing easier.*
*** Use clingfilm (plastic wrap) that contains no PVC as tuna is an oily fish. Also, roll or pound the fish gently or you will cause tears in the slices and ruin the final appearance of the dish. Use a cutlet bat or small wooden mallet.*

**** The julienne of horseradish should resemble strands of hair. If this effect is too difficult to achieve or fresh horseradish is not available, you can blend some bottled horseradish with 1–2 tablespoons of single cream (light cream) in the blender and drizzle this over the fish. The fresh horseradish shreds look best and give the most authentic flavour, however.*

Crispy-skinned Seabass (Striped Bass)with Flat-leaf Parsley (Italian Parsley) and Sorrel Salad

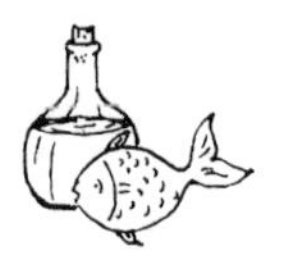

A great dish to serve on a hot summer's day, garnished with boiled Jersey Royals or other new potatoes. Exquisite!

This dish can be served as either a main course or a starter. As a starter, you need to allow a 75-g (3-oz) boneless seabass (striped bass) fillet per portion. Double this quantity for a main course.

This recipe is versatile in other ways, too, as it can be used for salmon, mullet and chicken!

With this simple recipe you can produce a fine dish, but success depends on timing and the use of excellent ingredients. Simple dishes *are* the best, but they must be prepared with thought and skill. Practice makes perfect!

*40 g (1½ oz) lambs' lettuce (corn salad)**
*40 g (1½ oz) leaves from the centre of a frisée lettuce (curly endive)***
50–75 g (2–3 oz) fresh sorrel
50–75 g (2–3 oz) fresh flat-leaf parsley (Italian parsley)
3 or 4 small sprigs of chervil
1 bunch of watercress
4 tbsp Flat-leaf Parsley (Italian Parsley) Oil (see page 11) or 4tbsp olive oil
juice of 1 lemon or a few drops of balsamic vinegar
4 seabass (striped bass) fillets, boned but with skin
1–2 tsp olive oil
2 tbsp Flat-leaf Parsley (Italian Parsley) Oil
4 tbsp Tomato Vinaigrette (see page 23)
sea salt

1. Prepare the salad and herbs by washing and drying the leaves. Dress with a combination of either olive oil and lemon juice or – my preference – a blend

of the 4 tablespoons of the Flat-leaf Parsley (Italian Parsley) Oil and a few drops of balsamic vinegar. The sweetness of the balsamic vinegar adds depth to the taste of the fish.

2. For the seabass (striped bass), sprinkle the fish with fine sea salt. I don't particularly like to season fish with pepper unless it is a flavour I want to emphasize in the dish.

3. Pour about 1 tsp of olive oil into a heavy-based *non-stick* frying pan and place over a high heat. Score the skin of the fish with a sharp knife to form crosses (this prevents the fish from curling during cooking). Place the pieces of fish – skin side down – in the hot pan and fry until the skin is crisp. At this point, you may find that there is quite a bit of smoke coming from the pan, but that is to be expected. The intensity of the heat is needed to crisp up the skin of the fish. The exact cooking time will depend on the size of the piece of fish. After 2–3 minutes, carefully flip over each piece and sprinkle the skin with a small amount of sea salt. You can tell when the fish is cooked by piercing the thickest part of the fish with a skewer. When the skewer meets no resistance whatsoever, the fish is cooked. Be sure not to overcook the fish. When cooked, remove the fish from the pan to a hot oven tray and place under a heated grill (broiler) for another 2–3 minutes.

4. Divide the dressed salad between 4 serving plates, then place a piece of fish, skin side up, on top of each mound of leaves. Trail the remaining Flat-leaf Parsley (Italian Parsley) Oil and Tomato Vinaigrette around the edge of each plate and serve.

** The mix of salad leaves is up to you, but I like using several soft herbs for this recipe. Basil and tarragon are a bit too strong, but flat-leaf parsley (Italian parsley), baby spinach, watercress and coriander go well with sorrel. Rocket (arugula), in small amounts, will also work.*

*** Use the soft, inner leaves of frisée (curly endive) for their texture and a colour contrast – the green outer leaves are too bitter for this dish. The frisée also gives some height to the salad.*

Hot-smoked Fillet of Wild Salmon

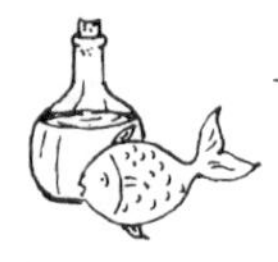

The great thing about hot-smoking food is that it is virtually fat free: the results are modern, light and truly delicious. Hot-smoking was once impossible in the average home, but recent interest in the technique has encouraged manufacturers to produce small and reasonably priced smoke boxes that give professional results. Prices and sizes vary, so shop around.

There is a vast difference between hot- and cold-smoked fish. The kind of smoked salmon enjoyed on a bagel with cream cheese is doused in brine and then, at a moderate temperature (45°C/113°F or below), exposed to wood smoke. Cold-smoking preserves food by killing bacteria and other micro-organisms, seals in moisture by slightly drying the outer flesh and adds the distinctive flavour of wood smoke. This produces the familiar slightly salty, soft, pink flesh we look for in good smoked salmon when we are planning a party. With a few exceptions – such as salmon – cold-smoked fish needs to be cooked before serving.

Even tastier, to my thinking, is hot-smoked salmon – a favourite in western Canada. Prepared in this way, the fish loses its pink, raw appearance and takes on a deeper, meatier flavour. That is the effect we want with this recipe.

Although the following recipe is for salmon, you can use the same technique for any oily fish and be proud of the finished dish. Tuna is excellent prepared this way, for example. Hot-smoked fish is a favourite with our guests at One Paston Place.

Serve your salmon on crispy fried Chinese noodles (see page 79) or as part of a light salad dressed with Tomato Vinaigrette (see page 23).

75 g (3 oz) of salmon fillet per person as a starter;
150–175 g (5–6 oz) for a main course

The size of the fish determines the length of time required for smoking (follow the manufacturer's instructions), but a 75-g (3-oz) fillet will take about 3–5 minutes, depending on how thick the piece of fish is. Generally, we keep the salmon a little bit underdone, so it remains a little pink in the middle. This is not to everyone's taste, but I strongly believe you should not overcook oily fish.

Crispy-skinned Wild Salmon with Rice Noodles

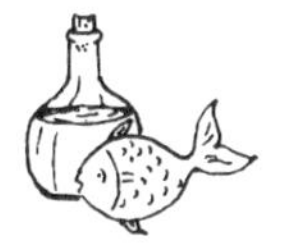

This is one of my favourite recipes – good flavour, nice appearance, very low fat content. A dish that sums up the essence of what this book is about – healthy eating with a modern touch.

Simple dishes require the finest ingredients so although you can use farmed salmon in this recipe, wild salmon gives better results. Also, if you serve farmed salmon with a sauce, it can mask the flavour of the fish, so you upset the balance of tastes you are trying to achieve.

The noodles are an easy way to add a nice touch to many dishes.

50 g (2 oz) vermicelli Chinese noodles
vegetable oil (not olive oil), for frying
4 x 75-g (3-oz) pieces of wild salmon, with skin
4 tbsp soy sauce
2 tbsp roasted sesame seed oil
8 tbsp Chinese-style Vinaigrette (see page 24)
1 tbsp sesame and poppy seeds
1 tbsp chopped spring onions (scallions)
1 tbsp chopped coriander leaves

1. Prepare the noodles by deep frying them in fresh oil at a temperature of 180°C/350°F for a very short period of time – they puff up very quickly. Remove at once and drain.

2. Marinate the pieces of fish in the soy sauce for 5 minutes, skin side down, ensuring that just the skin is in the soy sauce.*

3. When the fish has marinated, cut the skin shallowly crosswise several times with a sharp knife. This helps the heat penetrate quickly.

4. Pan-fry the wild salmon – skin side down – in the sesame seed oil for 3–4 minutes, or until the skin is quite black.

5. Flip the pieces of fish over and fry until cooked. You can tell when the salmon

is done by piercing the thickest part with a skewer; when the skewer meets no resistance, the fish is cooked.

6. Divide the deep-fried noodles equally between 4 plates. Arrange a piece of salmon on each, skin side up.
7. To finish, spoon 2 tablespoons of Chinese-style Vinaigrette around the edge of each pile of noodles and sprinkle some of the sesame and poppy seeds, spring onions (scallions) and coriander over the whole plate.

** The objective here is to darken the skin and add flavour. And, because the salt in the soy sauce will help draw water out of the skin, it enhances the crispyness of the finished dish. You want to achieve a contrast between the crispy skin and nice, moist salmon. Therefore it is important that the soy sauce should not touch the pink flesh of the fish because its taste can become overpowering, so limit the depth and amount of soy sauce you use.*

Mackerel Beignets

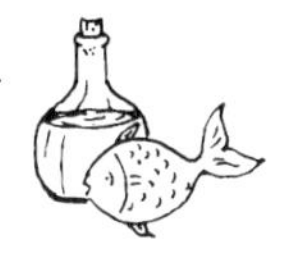

Mackerel is a popular fish throughout the North Atlantic region, where it is broiled, soused, smoked and fried. Using the fresh, firm flesh of the fish in beignets, or fritters, is a quick, modern way to take advantage of its delicious flavour and firm texture. A bonus is that mackerel is one of the oily fish that nutritionists recommend eating more of as they contain high levels of the omega–3 fatty acids, which are beneficial to our health.

4 x 350-g (12-oz) mackerel, filleted and bones removed
2 tbsp plain (all-purpose) flour, seasoned with salt and pepper
oil, for frying
1 quantity Rice Batter for Deep Frying (see page 44)
50 g (2 oz/2 cups) watercress leaves
50 g (2 oz) rocket (arugula)
25 g (1 oz) leaves from centre of frisée (curly endive)
2 tbsp extra virgin olive oil
a few drops 8-year-old balsamic vinegar
8 tbsp Tomato Vinaigrette (see page 23)
salt and freshly ground black pepper

1. Cut each fillet in half and season with salt and pepper.
2. Heat the oil in a fryer to 325–350°F/170–180°C.
3. Coat the mackerel fillets with the seasoned flour, then the batter and plunge into the hot oil. Fry until crisp and golden brown.* Drain the cooked fillets on paper kitchen towel.
4. Season the Mackerel Beignets lightly with salt and pepper.
5. Toss the salad leaves with the olive oil and balsamic vinegar and arrange on 4 plates. For this dish, form a mound – or dome – of leaves in the centre of each plate, leaving the edge clear for the fish.
6. Spoon a narrow ring of Tomato Vinaigrette around the salad and arrange the fish on the Vinaigrette. Serve immediately.

* *Obviously, cooking times will vary depending on the size of the fillets, but as a rough guide, normally, for mackerel weighing between 300 and 350 g (10 and 12 oz), you should find that 2–2½ minutes is adequate.*

Chinese-style Monkfish Ravioli

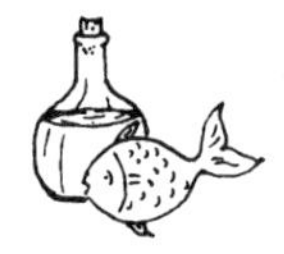

This is a fine starter or main course. Don't be put off by the long list of ingredients and instructions as it is a very simple dish to prepare and absolutely stunning.

1 medium squid, including the tentacles
2 tsp soy sauce
24 sheets of won ton pastry (approximately 8 cm/3¼ in square)
12 fresh coriander leaves, washed and dried, plus 1 tbsp chopped coriander
1 sheet Japanese nori seaweed, cut into 24 pieces each 1 cm/½ in square
100 g (4 oz) monkfish, cut into 12 equal pieces
1 egg yolk, beaten and thinned with a few drops of water
1 tbsp sesame oil
4 portions of deep-fried Chinese noodles (see page 79)
6 tbsp Chinese-style Vinaigrette (see page 24)
1 tbsp chopped spring onion (scallion)
1 tbsp poppy or sesame seeds, toasted
freshly ground black pepper

1. Cut the squid into 12 circular pieces and divide the tentacles into 4 portions. Marinate in the soy sauce with a little black pepper. Set to one side.
2. On a non-stick surface, such as baking parchment, lay out 12 sheets of the won ton pastry.
3. On top of each, place a coriander leaf and a square of Japanese nori seaweed.
4. Top each with a piece of monkfish.
5. Place a small square of nori on top of the fish.
6. Around the outside edge of each won ton, brush just a little of the thinned egg yolk.
7. Cover each won ton with another piece of pastry; press the edges down firmly to make a tight seal. Cover with clingfilm (plastic wrap) and put to one side.
8. Just before preparing the serving plates, cook the Monkfish Ravioli. Place

them in a steamer on a heatproof plate or dish that has been lightly brushed with a little of the sesame oil not touching each other. Cooking takes only 2–3 minutes. Because monkfish cooks very quickly and gets tough when it is overcooked, you want to keep an eye on the time. Remove them from the heat and set them on one side when done.

9. When the Monkfish Ravioli go into the steamer, heat the remaining sesame oil in a non-stick pan and quickly fry the marinated squid. Again, this will take very little time, so watch them carefully.
10. On each of 4 plates, place a small dome of deep-fried Chinese noodles, arrange 3 Monkfish Ravioli around them and top the noodles with the pieces of squid.
11. Slightly warm the Chinese-style Vinaigrette and add the chopped coriander leaves and spring onion. Spoon over the Monkfish Ravioli.
12. Sprinkle the plate with the toasted poppy or sesame seeds and serve to your guests.

Warm Scallop (Sea Scallop) and Langoustine (Jumbo Shrimp) Salad

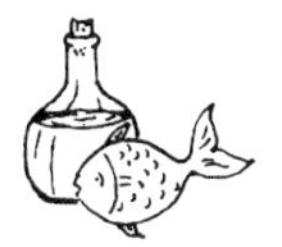

The Langoustine Oil used in this recipe takes time to prepare, so, if time is short, this delicious salad can be made by substituting warmed Tomato Vinaigrette (see page 23). However, it will taste quite different so do make time for the full recipe at some point in the future.

*4 large scallops (sea scallops)**
*3 langoustines (jumbo shrimp)***
4 tbsp Langoustine Oil (see page 19)
about 100 g (4 oz) mixed salad leaves
1 tbsp extra virgin olive oil
a few drops of balsamic vinegar
25 g (1 oz/⅔ cup) chopped chives
sea salt and freshly ground black pepper

1. Just before preparing this dish, slice each scallop (sea scallop) into three coin-shaped pieces.
2. Shell the langoustines. For each, remove the head. Then, holding the top (head end) of the langoustine between your thumb and forefinger, squeeze gently until the shell cracks. Peel off the first top sections of shell and then squeeze the tail end gently until the flesh pops out of the shell. (Peeling shrimp is much easier.) You can use the shell to make Langoustine Oil (see page 19). (You cannot use shrimp shells to make Langoustine Oil.)
3. Place 1 tablespoon of the Langoustine Oil in a non-stick pan and heat. Quickly fry the langoustines (jumbo shrimp) for 1½–2 minutes. Season with salt and pepper. Remove from the frying pan and keep warm.
4. At the very last minute, heat 1 tablespoon of Langoustine Oil and quickly fry the scallops (sea scallops) for 30 seconds on each side – if you cook them any longer than this they will become very tough.

5. Toss the salad leaves with the olive oil and balsamic vinegar and arrange on 4 plates.
6. Warm the remaining Langoustine Oil. Add a few drops of balsamic vinegar and the chives.
7. Arrange the scallops (sea scallops) and langoustines (jumbo shrimp) around the salad. Drizzle the warmed Langoustine Oil mixture around the edges of the plates – its beautiful orange-red colour makes a fantastic contrast with the soft colours of the salad leaves and shellfish – and serve immediately.

** What is a large scallop (sea scallop)? On the market today are scallops (sea scallops) in shells 15–18 cm/6–7 in across – the best of these caught by divers rather than being pulled up by dredgers. Although they are expensive, these are the ones you want to buy because they are the highest quality. The diver-caught scallops are hand picked off the bottom of the sea; dredged scallops are dragged along in nets by trawlers. During the dredging, the shellfish pick up lots of sand and dirt that must be carefully washed away before they can be cooked, which can take a considerable amount of time. Also, have your fishmonger open the shells and remove the muscle from each.*

*** Langoustines are sold by size and described by the number of them to a kilogram (2¼ lbs). For example, if the number is 21/30, you'll get between 21 and 30 in a kilo. For this dish, the 21/30 give a satisfactory result, but the 16/20s are a bit more generous.*

Light meats

Chicken, duck, quail and rabbit are excellent meats for healthy eating. Light and delicious, they can be made as formal or informal as you wish.

Duck Confit

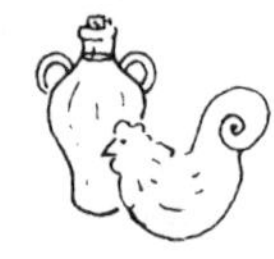

Although duck confit is available in jars and cans and may be purchased fresh, making your own is a rewarding experience and results in a better product.

In rural France, preparing confit is a method of preserving food that has been used for countless generations. Each week during the summer, farmers select one or two of their best ducks for Sunday's main meal. The livers are preserved in rendered duck fat for the Christmas season and the tender breasts – the choicest meat – is prepared for the meal. The legs and other bits and pieces of flesh from the carcase are not thrown away but made into a terrine for use later in the year, so nothing is wasted.

I enjoy serving this Duck Confit salad at One Paston Place and it is very popular with our guests. You can use the same basic technique I use to prepare duck legs at the restaurant to prepare confit at home for your own dinner table. Breaking with the rules, instead of giving you a recipe, I am going to 'talk' you through the process.

I buy fresh duck legs. To begin, I place them in a large container and sprinkle them heavily with sea salt – 1 tablespoon of salt per leg is about right. This draws the blood out of the meat and improves its flavour. Next, I add cracked black pepper, a favourite ingredient of mine, and some thyme, which complements the taste of duck. All this is left in the refrigerator for 24 hours.

Then, I wash the salt and herbs off and place the duck legs in a deep roasting tin and cover them completely with rendered duck fat.* I then place the tin in a 150°C/300°F/gas 2 oven and leave it to cook for about 3 hours, or until the meat will separate from the bones when moved.

I then take the duck out of the pan and allow it to cool. When cool, I put the duck legs into a clean jar and cover it completely with the melted fat from the pan, leave it to cool, then screw the lid on tightly.

The result is a very simple, traditional dish – duck cooked in its own fat. Sounds terrible, doesn't it? But it truly is delicious; particularly when you balance the richness of the meat with sharp, contrasting flavours of fruit or wine.

When preparing duck leg salad in the restaurant, I begin by slightly warming a piece – enough to remove any excess fat as it then drains off on paper kitchen towel – dusting the skin with icing sugar (confectioner's sugar) and placing it under a very hot grill (broiler). This makes a glaze on the meat that enhances its appearance and adds the pleasant contrast of caramelized sugar to the taste. Then, I lay the duck on a crisp salad of mixed leaves, dressed with a few drops of good-quality balsamic vinegar and a little pistachio or walnut oil. Finally, around the outside of the salad, I drop just two or three little dribbles of pistachio oil** – which is a clear and appetizing forest green. The result is a combination of sweet and salty, crisp and soft, plus fresh and cooked: a dish with contrasts to remember.

** You can use fresh or canned duck or goose fat. In France, these ingredients are reasonably priced, but elsewhere it may be cheaper to make your own. When you next roast a duck, try putting water in the bottom of the pan to save the fat from burning. The fat rendered during roasting can be drawn off once the duck has cooked. It usually has a pleasant, slightly roasted flavour. Alternatively, you can simply pull out the fatty deposits from inside an uncooked duck, place them in a saucepan, cover with water and simmer for an hour. Skim off the fat and store it in the refrigerator for use later. You can also use the entire duck for confit. This results in a good quantity of rendered fat for baking and storing the confit, but I prepare only the legs because they have the best flavour and texture.*

*** The pistachio oil has a good colour, but you can use any of the nut oils; they all go nicely with duck. Try walnut or hazelnut, for example. Which oil you use is a matter of personal preference, but I think it is best to avoid walnut oil which tastes too much of walnut shell, which is bitter and does not complement the sweetness of the duck. Also, you want to use something other than olive oil. Although duck with olives is a traditional, classic dish, for today's tastes, it is a little too heavy and there is not enough of a contrast between the oil from the plant and the fat in the duck meat.*

CONFIT TREATS

Duck confit is very versatile. For a main course, try serving it with sweet potatoes, bubble and squeak or braised red cabbage and apples dressed with cider vinegar. Alternatively, for something oriental, add it to stir-fried vegetables or wrap some confit in egg roll skins and serve them as spring rolls. For a beautiful starter, mix the duck meat with a little cooked and drained spinach, add some sautéd wild mushrooms, season to taste, wrap in filo pastry, brush with walnut oil and bake in a 150°C/300°F/gas 2 oven for about 20 minutes, or until golden brown.

Quail and Green Bean Salad with Walnut Oil Dressing

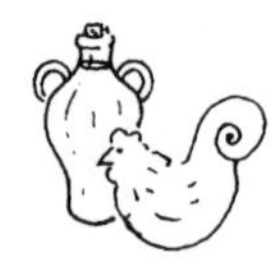

Although small, quail have enormous appeal because of their splendid taste and low fat content. This dish requires more effort and detailed preparation than most recipes in this book, but I think you will find the extra work to be worth while.

4 quail
1 tsp sea salt
225 g (8 oz) extra fine green beans
4 tbsp goose or duck fat (canned or rendered at home)
2 tbsp neutral-flavoured vegetable oil (such as grapeseed or sunflower), plus extra for frying
1 tsp finely chopped shallots
1 tbsp Walnut Oil Dressing (see page 29)
4 quails' eggs
4 tbsp Sharp Red Wine and Walnut Oil Vinaigrette (see page 26)
1 tbsp chopped chives
sea salt and freshly ground black pepper

1. The day before you plan to prepare this salad, choose the quail and have the butcher remove the legs for you.*
2. Season the legs with the measured quantity of sea salt. Place in a shallow dish, cover with clingfilm (plastic wrap) and leave in the refrigerator for 2–4 hours.
3. Meantime, begin preparing the green beans. Top and tail the beans and blanch in boiling water. Continue to cook until the beans are done, but still have a slight crunch; 4–5 minutes should be adequate. Refresh in cold water and set aside.
4. Preheat the oven to 150°C/300°F/gas 2.
5. After the 4 hours, rinse the salt off the quail legs, pat them dry with paper kitchen towel and place in a deep ovenproof dish.

6. Cover the legs with the goose or duck fat and place in the preheated oven for approximately 30 minutes. Remove them from the oven and turn it up to 220°C/425°F/gas 7.
7. Remove the legs from the fat and place them on an ovenproof tray. Season the quail breast portions with salt and pepper, place – with the vegetable oil – in a roasting tin and bake in the hotter oven for 4–5 minutes.
8. Remove the quail breasts from the oven and let them relax – skin side down – for 5–6 minutes.
9. Grill (broil) the quail legs for 3 minutes.
10. When they have cooled, carefully remove the breast meat from the bones. The goal is to obtain 2 intact portions of breast meat for each salad.
11. When it is time to arrange the salad on the plates, pour boiling water over the beans to warm them then drain them well.
12. Toss the beans with the shallots and Walnut Oil Dressing and season to taste with salt and pepper.
13. Place a small bundle of seasoned green beans in the centre of each of 4 plates. Lay half a quail breast each side of the green beans and place the quail legs in the gaps between.
14. In a small, non-stick pan, lightly fry the quails' eggs in a little vegetable oil and then place an egg on top of each bundle of green beans.
15. Dress the salad by spooning 1 tablespoon of Sharp Red Wine and Walnut Vinaigrette around the outer edge of the quail.
16. Finish with a sprinkling of chopped chives.

** If you want to make use of the quail carcases, place them in a pan with a little vegetable oil and fry over a high heat for 3–4 minutes. Drain off the excess oil, cover with chicken stock or water, bring to the boil and cook for 10 minutes. Strain the liquid through muslin (cheesecloth), then return it to the pan. Cook down until the sauce has the consistency of a light syrup. Spoon this carefully around the edges of the quail salad.*

Skinless Grilled (Broiled) Chicken Breast with Mushroom Tapenade and Savoy Cabbage

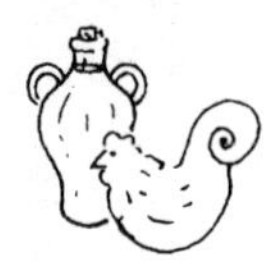

This is a simple dish that – when executed perfectly – can make even the sternest dinner guest smile.

To add contrast to the plate, you could serve this dish with Deep-fried Root Vegetables (see page 54).

1 good-sized Savoy cabbage
4 free-range, corn-fed or poulet noire chicken breasts
(about 200–225g/7–8 oz after the skin has been removed)
6 tbsp Mushroom Tapenade (see page 41)
*a few drops of truffle oil**
6 tbsp Mushroom Oil (see page 17)
a few drops of 8-year-old balsamic vinegar
1 tbsp chopped chives
sea salt and freshly ground black pepper

1. Preheat the oven to 200°C/400°F/gas 7.
2. Prepare the cabbage. Remove the outside leaves, cut the cabbage into quarters and remove the core from each.
3. Cut the cabbage into strips – about 1 by 5 cm (½ by 2 in) – and rinse with cold water.
4. Plunge the cabbage into boiling salted water for 2 minutes.
5. Pour the cabbage into a colander and leave to drain, but do not rinse with cold water. Cabbage tends to hold water and, at this point, you want to remove as much fluid as possible from the cabbage without damaging its texture.
6. Season the chicken breasts well with salt and pepper.

7. On a *hot* grill,** place the chicken pieces best side – or presentation side – down and leave to cook.
8. After 3–4 minutes, give each chicken breast a quarter turn and, with a bit of luck, you should have a nice criss-cross pattern when the chicken is finished. Leave to cook another 3–4 minutes.
9. Turn the breast pieces over and repeat the process.
10. Remove the chicken from the grill and bake in the preheated oven for 6–7 minutes.
11. When the chicken is cooked,*** remove it from the oven and let it stand on a warm plate for a further 4–5 minutes. This allows the meat to 'rest'.****
12. While the chicken breasts are relaxing, heat the Mushroom Tapenade (you can make this 1–2 days before).
13. Back to the Savoy cabbage. Using your hands, gently squeeze out the remaining moisture. Place the cabbage in a microwave dish, season with salt and pepper, cover with clingfilm (plastic wrap) and warm through in a 650-watt microwave for 20 seconds. Alternatively, put a tablespoon of water in a non-stick pan with the cabbage, cover the pan and cook over a moderate heat for 3 minutes or until the cabbage is heated through thoroughly.
14. When the cabbage is warm, sprinkle with a few drops of the truffle oil. Check the seasoning and keep warm until ready to serve.
15. On 4 warm plates, place a good spoonful of the warmed Mushroom Tapenade. Slice the chicken breasts into 2 or 3 pieces and place on top of the Tapenade. Next to the chicken, spoon a dome, or neat mound, of the Savoy cabbage. Surround the whole plate with a drizzle of Mushroom Oil and a few spots of 8-year-old balsamic vinegar. Sprinkle with chopped chives and serve.

> * *Good truffle oil can be purchased from many delicatessens (Italian grocers and gourmet food stores). It is quite expensive, but a little goes a long way, so it is worth buying. It is truly excellent on cabbage.*
>
> ** *By grilling here I mean charcoal grilling – almost barbecuing – so the grill must be very hot. The grills you use must be spotlessly clean. You can buy all sorts of grill brushes these days, so buy one you like and make sure it is well used.*

**** It is imperative that the chicken is cooked through, but still moist. In France, they call it moellux, which means moist. There is nothing worse than a piece of dried up old chicken, but few things better than a piece of moist, good-quality, freshly cooked chicken. Grilling chicken, like anything else in cooking, takes a little time and a little experience before you get it just right. To see whether or not the chicken is cooked, pierce the thickest part with a skewer and if you meet very little resistance going through, it is cooked. The best way to experience what this resistance feels like is to push a skewer through a chicken breast before you cook it. You will then immediately understand what I mean by 'resistance' and, likewise, when you test it after cooking know what I mean when I say that the skewer meets very little resistance. It is all a matter of feel.*

***** It is important to let the chicken rest, or relax, for 4–5 minutes after cooking. Most people forget that the juices in meats need time to settle. Remembering this simple fact can make the difference between a tough and tender final product.*

Rabbit Salad with Fresh Peas and Broad Beans (Fava Beans)

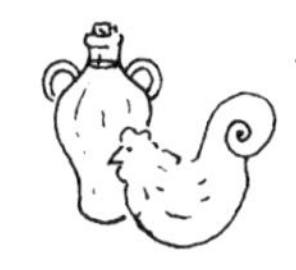

The nutritious and appetizing blend of ingredients in this salad make it a hit as a starter or main course.

If you are looking for low-fat alternatives to more traditional meats, I suggest you try rabbit. Buy the best and freshest you can find, and only from a reputable source.

At the restaurant, we buy whole rabbits and use the legs in confit, which is then served with polenta or as a salad. Ask your butcher to prepare the carcases for you.*

While it may seem like a lot of work making the confit, it really is not. Just allow adequate time to completely cook the meat and you will be rewarded with a beautiful meal.

saddles and shoulders of 2 rabbits
2 tsp sea salt
225 g(8 oz/1 cup) goose or duck fat (canned or rendered at home)
1 tbsp vegetable oil
250 g (9 oz) freshly shelled and cooked peas
150 g (5 oz) freshly cooked broad beans (fava beans)
75 g (3 oz) extra fine green beans, cut into 5-mm/¼-in lengths
1 tsp finely diced shallots
2 tbsp Walnut Oil Dressing (see page 29)
*2 tbsp hazelnut or walnut oil***
sea salt and freshly ground black pepper

1. Prepare the rabbit, making a confit from the 4 shoulder sections in the following way. The day before you plan to serve this dish, liberally sprinkle the 4 shoulder pieces with the 2 teaspoons of sea salt and leave them in the refrigerator for 5–6 hours.
2. Preheat the oven to 110°C/225°F/gas ¼.
3. Rinse off the salt, place the meat in a deep bowl and cover completely with the melted goose or duck fat. Bake in the preheated oven for 1½–2

hours, or until the meat easily separates from the bones. This can be done well ahead of time. Then, turn the oven up to 200°C/400°F/gas 6.

4. Heat the vegetable oil in a heavy-based frying pan. Season the 2 rabbit saddles with salt and pepper and fry for about 2–3 minutes on each side. Remove from the pan, place them on a baking sheet and bake in the hotter oven for 8–10 minutes. Remove the meat from the oven, leave the oven on, and allow the meat to rest for 4–5 minutes.
5. Meanwhile, prepare the vegetables for the salad. Plunge the peas, broad beans (fava beans) and green beans into boiling salted water for 30 seconds, then tip them into a colander to drain off the water. Place the drained vegetables in a bowl and add the chopped shallots and Walnut Oil Dressing. Mix them together gently with a spoon.
6. Divide the cooked and dressed vegetables between 4 plates.
7. Reheat the rabbit confit (the shoulders) in the oven for 3 minutes.
8. Meanwhile, remove the long strips of meat – the loin – from the saddle sections with a sharp knife.*** Slice each of these deliciously tender morsels into 6 pieces and arrange around the vegetables. Two saddles should provide 12 pieces, or 3 slices, per serving.
9. Remove the confit from the oven and use paper kitchen towel to remove any excess fat. Place the confit on top of the vegetables. Warm the hazelnut or walnut oil and drizzle a little around the edge of each plate. The rabbit liver and kidneys can be added to the salad if you wish. Simply cut each in half and sauté in a little vegetable oil for 2–3 minutes.

** The rabbit carcase can be used to make a sauce to spoon around the salad. See page 90 and simply substitute the rabbit for the quail.*

*** I enjoy using roasted rapeseed oil (toasted canola seed oil) when making this dish at One Paston Place. However, it is difficult to obtain and unrefined nut oils are equally good with the meat.*

**** Removing the cooked loin from the saddle sections is quite easy. Place the rabbit saddle, ribs pointing up, on a chopping board and, using a sharp knife, cut along the ribs straight down towards the backbone. As soon as you hit the backbone, angle the knife to the right or to the left, and then lift the loin – the eye of the meat – away from the ribs.*

Accompaniments

Fats add much to simple vegetable dishes. They enrich the sensation of a food in the mouth and add an appealing sheen to its surface. A surprising amount of butter or margarine can disappear into a bowl of mashed potatoes or puréed root vegetables, though, and a simple bowl of green beans needs at least one good knob (pat) of butter to achieve a glossy, finished appearance.

One of the nice things about cooking with oils, however, is that they are equally good at enriching the sensation of taste and adding a gloss to vegetables, but you need less oil than butter or margarine to achieve the same effect. Instead of the usual generous portion of butter or cream I once used in purées, I find that a much smaller quantity of nut oil enhances the texture of these vegetables and adds significantly to their flavour. Also, I like the way in which the natural flavours of certain oils blend with vegetables.

Although they may be difficult to find and more expensive, unrefined, roasted nut oils carry the biggest taste 'punch'. Try hazelnut oil with pumpkin, for example or, as given in one recipe in this section, with parsnips.

Parsnip and Hazelnut Oil Purée

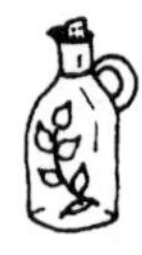

This tasty purée goes well with roast chicken, rabbit, quail and game.

400 g (14 oz) peeled parsnips (cores removed)*
3 tbsp hazelnut oil
large pinch of freshly grated nutmeg
salt and freshly ground black pepper

1. Place the prepared parsnips in boiling salted water and cook about 20 minutes, or until tender.
2. Drain the cooked parsnips in a colander and leave to cool for about 5 minutes.
3. Either mash together by hand or puree in a blender the parsnips, hazelnut oil and nutmeg.
4. Add salt and pepper to taste and serve.

** It is important to remove the tough cores from the parsnips because they detract from the smoothness of the purée.*

Crushed Potato with Spring Onions (Scallions) and Flat-leaf Parsley (Italian Parsley)

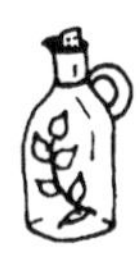

Altering the texture of a dish can change its entire character and appeal. This simple method for preparing potatoes differs from others because the vegetables are gently crushed with a fork, not beaten or mashed into a purée. I find that guests at One Paston Place ask for the recipe and when I explain how easy it is, many suggest I must have left out some vital, secret ingredient. There are no secrets, though – just follow these simple instructions and use good-quality potatoes. We find that the best potatoes for this are the old-fashioned variety Pink Fir Apple and Roseval. We also use Charlotte and the French variety Belle de Fontenay. If none of these is available, use a variety that has a firm texture when cooked.

Young helpers in the kitchen will find that this is a satisfyingly easy dish to make for the family.

approximately 700 g (1½ lbs) firm potatoes (see above)
4 spring onions (scallions)
2 tbsp flat-leaf parsley (Italian parsley)
*2–4 tbsp extra virgin olive oil**
sea salt and freshly ground black pepper

1. Place the potatoes in a pan of cold water with a good teaspoon of sea salt. Bring to the boil and simmer for 20 minutes, or until cooked.**

2. While the potatoes are cooking, coarsely chop the spring onions (scallions) and flat-leaf parsley (Italian parsley). You want to create a bit of texture and colour in this dish, so keep the pieces of parsley fairly large.

3. When the potatoes have cooled, peel them and put them into a large bowl.

4. Add the spring onions (scallions) and parsley.

5. Crush, or break up the cooked potatoes with a fork.

6. Gently mix the olive oil into the vegetables.

** The amount of oil you will need really depends on your choice of potatoes. Obviously, you do not want the final dish to be too greasy, so add a little at a time until you get the consistency you want. The oil is there to bring out the best in the texture and flavour of the potatoes, not overwhelm them.*

*** The easiest way to tell if the potatoes are cooked is to push a sharp, pointed knife into one of the largest in the pot and lift it out of the water – when the potato slips off the knife easily, the potatoes are done.*

Provençal Vegetables with Pistou

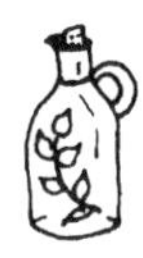

Provençal Vegetables with Pistou is rather like ratatouille, but with a richer taste. It can be served with rice as a vegetarian dish or served as an accompaniment for fish. The flavour and texture of cod, red mullet (red snapper), seabass (striped bass), monkfish and hake are all balanced nicely by this combination of ingredients. Try it with roast chicken or leg of lamb – it is very good with these. Use this recipe, too, as the foundation for a classic French dish, Soupe au Pistou. You will find a recipe for this hearty main-course soup on page 60.

This dish should be finished just before serving, but all of the vegetables can be prepared well ahead of time.

1 large red pepper (bell pepper)
1 small yellow pepper (bell pepper)
2–3 tbsp extra virgin olive oil
1 medium aubergine (eggplant)
1 bulb fennel
4 medium courgettes (zucchini)
3 tablespoons Pistou (see page 38)
12 Tomato Petals (see page 32)
½ cup Fennel Stock (see page 46)
2 tbsp pine nuts, toasted
sea salt and freshly ground black pepper

1. Brush the peppers with some of the olive oil and place on a baking sheet under a very hot grill (broiler). Turn the vegetables when their skins begin to blister.
2. When the peppers are blistered all over, remove them from the grill (broiler) and place in a bowl or air-tight container. Cover with clingfilm (plastic wrap) or lid and leave for 10–12 minutes.
3. Remove the peppers from the bowl or container and hold them under a running cold water tap (faucet). The skins should lift off easily and can be removed with a knife.
4. Cut the peeled peppers into quarters, remove the seeds and the centre core,

and cut them into pieces about 1 cm (½ in) square. Put to one side.

5. Wipe and cut the aubergine (eggplant) into 1-cm (½-in) dice. Put to one side.*

6. Prepare the courgettes (zucchini) by first removing their watery central core, which tends to go very soft when cooked. To do this, place a courgette on its side and, using a sharp knife, slice off a section about a third of the way in from one side. Turn the courgette (zucchini) over, laying it on the cut surface, and repeat the slicing process. This time, however, you will be able to see the seeds and be able to slice the tasty portion of the vegetable away cleanly from the watery core. Repeat until the core has been has been separated from the rest of the courgette (zucchini) and discard it. Dice the side sections of the courgette (zucchini).

7. Cut the tops off the fennel and chop the bulb into quarters, take out the core and dice the rest as before.

8. Place the diced aubergine (eggplant) in a heated non-stick pan. Season it with salt and pepper and cook over a fairly high heat without any oil whatsoever.** When the aubergine (eggplant) is cooked, remove it from the heat and place in a bowl or container.

9. Meanwhile, place the fennel in a saucepan of cold water and bring to the boil and simmer for 2 minutes.Then, drain and set aside.

10. Heat 1 tablespoon of the olive oil in a pan and sauté the courgettes (zucchini) and fennel, stirring occasionally.

11. Place the Pistou in a mortar with the Tomato Petals and crush to form a smooth paste.

12. Just before serving, bring the Fennel Stock to the boil and reduce by a third. Gently stir in the cooked vegetables. Bring back to the boil and cook for another 2 minutes.

13. Remove the pan from the heat and stir in the Pistou mixture. Add salt and pepper to taste.

14. Pour the vegetables into a serving dish, drizzle the remaining olive oil over and top with the toasted pine nuts. Serve immediately.

** When combining vegetables in a recipe, cut everything into pieces that are approximately the same size. The size recommended here – 1-cm (½-in) dice – gives a good appearance and texture to this dish.*

*** Aubergine (eggplant) is notorious for soaking up huge amounts of oil. However, I have found that the best way to avoid this problem is to prepare them dry. Also, some people sprinkle sliced sections with salt, allow them to drain and then rinse them before frying, but, in my opinion, whether this really makes a better end-product is questionable. By placing the chopped aubergine (eggplant) in a hot pan and stirring from time to time as the surfaces brown, the need for oil can be eliminated and the excess moisture is driven off. The amount of aubergine (eggplant) called for in this recipe should take 3–4 minutes to cook in this way.*

Sweet afters

Dessert is a happily anticipated part of a good meal. Unfortunately, many popular sweet 'afters' are laden with some form of saturated fat – usually cream or ice-cream. Even that favourite of many health-conscious eaters, carrot cake, is usually topped with a frosting made with cream cheese.

When it came to writing this section of the book, I wanted to include recipes that are light and healthy to counter this tendency. At the same time, I was looking for something modern in the way of cakes and biscuits (cookies). I hope you will agree that the following dishes meet these criteria.

In addition to being low in saturated fat, several of the recipes take advantage of the pleasing tastes and texture of nuts – particularly walnuts. From a nutritional standpoint, these are excellent additions to a meal because walnuts are rich in vitamins, minerals and essential fatty acids.

Melon with Honey and Lime

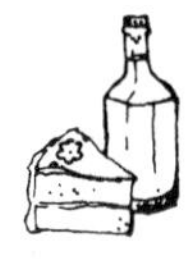

Here is a simple, zero-fat fruit dish guests at One Paston Place enjoy either as a starter or dessert. Its pastel colours and contrasting textures make this a fine dish for warm summer evenings.

SERVES 3

*2 small, ripe melons**
2 tbsp honey
juice of 2 limes
3 sprigs of fresh mint, the leaves finely sliced, or a few strands of Lime Confit (see page 106), to garnish
3 small bunches of redcurrants, to garnish

1. Cut the melons in half, remove the seeds, and halve again.
2. Slice each melon quarter into 3 equal slices and cut away the rind. You now have 24 slices.
3. On each of 3 plates, arrange, in the shape of a flower, 4 slices of both varieties of melon. Chill in the refrigerator.
4. Puree the remaining slices of the melon in a blender and press through a strainer.
5. Place the honey in a small saucepan and bring to the boil.
6. Add the lime juice and melon to the honey, remove the pan from the heat, strain, let it cool, then place in the refrigerator. It is imperative that the sauce and melon be well chilled before you use them.
7. When you are ready to serve the melon, spoon some of the honey and juice mixture around each dessert plate and garnish with a sprinkling of either julienne of mint or Lime Confit. Tuck the redcurrants beside a slice of melon for a touch of contrast.

* *If possible, combine a Galia melon – which has a fresh green centre*

– and a pinky-orange-fleshed Cantaloupe. The contrasting colours and textures add to the total pleasure of this dish.

Lime Confit

In the restaurant, we often use a confit of lime, orange or lemon and I am sure you will find many uses for it too. These glazed, highly flavoured strands can be used to enhance many different kinds of desserts.

To make it, you simply peel the zest from the fruit and cut it into very fine julienne strips before preparing as described below. For a professional appearance, cut the strips as finely as possible – almost like hairs. If you find this difficult, use a zester. This gadget produces strips that are not as fine as I like them, but it makes the task much easier and the finished confit is still very good. If you are peeling and cutting the zest, though, you want to make certain that all the white pith is removed because it is bitter and detracts from the clean taste of the fruit.

zest of 2 limes, prepared as described above
2 tbsp sugar

1. Place the lime strips in a saucepan with 2 tablespoons of water and bring to the boil.

2. Drain off the water, then add the sugar and just enough water to cover the julienne. Bring to the boil, then turn down the heat as low as possible, cover and simmer for about 1 hour. Check from time to time to make sure the water has not evaporated and left the sugar to burn.

3. When the strips are translucent, turn them out onto a non-stick surface and separate them so that they dry without sticking together.

Apple Strudel

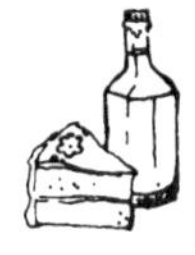

Baked fruit is an excellent way to end a meal. When it is wrapped in filo pastry and the texture level turned up with some nuts and raisins, you just forget that it contains very little fat and is packed with nutrients. This easy recipe makes every dinner a party.

Serve this easy and attractive dessert warm with low-fat fromage frais (fromage blanc).

4 Granny Smith apples (or other large, firm apples – Russets or Sturmer Pippins, for example)
50 g (2 oz/generous ¼ cup) brown sugar
25 g (1 oz/½ cup) dry breadcrumbs or cake crumbs
25 g (1 oz/scant ¼ cup) sultanas
25 g (1 oz/scant ¼ cup) raisins
25 g (1 oz/⅓ cup) ground almonds
25 g (1 oz/⅓ cup) flaked (slivered) almonds
zest and juice of ½ lemon
small pinch of ground mixed spice (apple pie spice)
4 sheets filo pastry (40 by 40 cm/15¾ by 15¾ in)
1 tbsp grilled almond or unrefined almond oil with a strong, nutty flavour
icing sugar (confectioners' sugar), for dusting

1. Preheat the oven to 200°C/400°F/gas 6.
2. Peel, core and quarter the apples. Cut each quarter into 5 or 6 pieces.
3. Place the apple pieces in a bowl, add the other ingredients, except the filo pastry and almond oil, and mix thoroughly.
4. Spread out the sheets of filo pastry and brush with some almond oil.
5. Place a small mound of apple mixture in the centre of each sheet of filo and fold the pastry over the mixture to form triangular, handkerchief-shaped packets, approximately the size of a man's clenched fist. Place on an oiled baking sheet and brush the outsides of the packets with almond oil and dust

liberally with icing sugar (confectioners' sugar). The sugar will produce a nice glaze during baking.

6. Bake in the preheated oven for 20 minutes.

VARIATION

You can use this same recipe to make an apricot strudel. Simply substitute 12 golf ball-size fresh apricots for the apples, increase the amount of sugar you use to 175 g (6 oz/scant cup) and leave out the lemon juice. Also, reduce the baking time to 10 minutes, or until they are golden brown.

Glazed Fennel and Walnut Cake

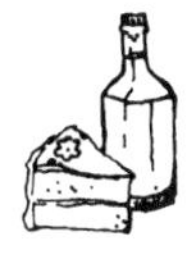

This updated version of the classic carrot cake has a surprisingly light taste that works well after a hearty winter meal of soup and salad. Make it the day before as this beauty improves with a little age!

MAKES ONE 20-CM/8-IN OR SIX 10-CM/4-IN CAKES

225 g (8 oz/generous 1½ cups) wholemeal (wholewheat) flour, sifted
1 tsp baking powder
1 tsp ground mixed spice (apple pie spice)
1½ tsp ground star anise
pinch of salt
175 g (6 oz/1 cup) finely grated fresh fennel bulb
150 g (5 oz/generous ⅓ cup) plus 1 tbsp brown sugar
175 g (2 oz/½ cup) walnuts, chopped
2 medium (large) eggs
115 ml (4 fl oz/½ cup) good-quality walnut oil
125 ml (4½ fl oz/generous ½ cup) fresh orange juice
finely cut zest of 1 orange
juice of 2 oranges
low-fat fromage frais (fromage blanc), to serve

1. Preheat the oven to 180°C/350°F/gas 4 and oil and lightly flour the cake tin, or tins, you are going to use.
2. Sift the flour, baking powder, spices and salt into a bowl.
3. Add the fennel, 150 g (5 oz/generous ⅓ cup) brown sugar and walnuts. Gently mix everything together.
4. In a separate bowl, whisk the eggs for 2 minutes, then continue whisking and add the oil and orange juice.
5. Slowly stir the flour mixture into the egg and oil mixture until well blended.

6. Tip the mixture into the prepared cake tin or divide it equally between the 4 small tins and bake in the centre of the preheated oven. A 20-cm/8-in cake should take about 1 hour; the 10-cm/4-in cakes will require 20–25 minutes. The cake or cakes are done when a skewer inserted into the centre comes out clean.
7. After baking, invert the cake or cakes onto a cooling rack and leave to cool.
8. Next, prepare the glaze. Begin by blanching the orange zest. To do this, place it in a saucepan with enough cold water to cover, bring it to the boil and cook for about 2 minutes, or until the skin begins to turn translucent.
9. Drain the water from the pan, then add the orange juice and remaining brown sugar. Place over a low heat and reduce until 3 tablespoons of liquid remain. Pour into a small bowl and leave to cool; the mixture will become thick.
10. Spoon the glaze over the cake or cakes and serve with low-fat fromage frais (fromage blanc).

Hazelnut Biscuits (Cookies)

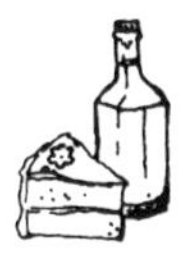

In keeping with our theme of healthy eating, this recipe contains no saturated fat and only a small amount of oil.

You can use this recipe in one of two ways. As small, bite-sized dropped biscuits (cookies) they are excellent with tea or an after-dinner coffee. However, if you smooth out the batter on a non-stick surface or baking parchment and make very thin biscuits (cookies), or disks, they can be used to create elegant desserts. They resemble a hazelnut mille-feuille. Simply place a thin biscuit (cookie) in the centre of a plate, cover it with fruit (poached pears glazed with caramel sauce or strawberries and fresh mango are good flavour combinations) and top with a second thin biscuit (cookie). A sprinkling of icing sugar (confectioners' sugar) on top – or, if you are in party mood, a tablespoon of whipped cream – produces a memorable end to a meal.

MAKES 6 ORDINARY OR 12 THIN BISCUITS (COOKIES)

175 g (6 oz/2 cups) ground hazelnuts or almonds
75 g (3 oz/generous ½ cup) icing sugar (confectioners' sugar), plus extra for dusting
75 g (3 oz/generous ½ cup) caster sugar (granulated sugar)
2½ tbsp stock syrup or sweet white wine*
1 tbsp honey
2 egg whites
2 tsp hazelnut oil, or almond oil if you are using ground almonds

1. Preheat the oven to 190°C/375°F/gas 5 and place all the ingredients in a bowl and leave in warm place for 30 minutes.

2. Mix well by hand. You should now have a thick paste. If the batter needs thinning at this point, add a touch more stock syrup or sweet white wine.

3. To make biscuits (cookies), place coffee spoon-sized mounds of the mixture on a non-stick baking sheet or one lined with baking parchment. Dampen each mound slightly with water using a pastry brush and dust with icing sugar (confectioners' sugar). Bake in the preheated oven for about 15 minutes.

4. To make the thin hazelnut *mille-feuille,* you need to cut some templates so that you end up with circular biscuits of equal size. A good way to do this is to begin by cutting 12 circles – about 4 cm/1½ in across – from non-stick parchment paper. Place a spoonful of the biscuit mixture in the centre of each circle and smooth it out evenly to the paper's edge. Bake at the same temperature as the ordinary biscuits (cookies), but watch them carefully – because they are very thin they tend to cook very quickly. When they have browned, lift the *mille-feuille* off their templates with a pallet knife and place them on a non-stick surface to cool. Try keeping a few on hand in an air-tight container for an easy, but sumptuous, ending to an impromptu dinner party.
5. To arrange the *mille-feuille,* allow 3 biscuits (cookies) for each portion and sandwich your favourite filling between them. Make certain you are not too generous with the filling or the biscuits (cookies) will crumble. When you are rushing to finish the dessert for your guests, this is not a welcome event! Dust with icing sugar (confectioners' sugar). The list of possible combinations for fillings is endless, but I suggest you try roasted peaches with caramel sauce or fresh berries mixed with fromage frais (fromage blanc). Whatever you try, keep the filling fairly dry and the pieces of fruit small and lightweight.

** To make stock syrup, place 2 tablespoons of water and 2 tablespoons of caster sugar (granulated sugar) in a saucepan and boil the mixture for 2 minutes. Leave it to cool before using.*

Afterword: Questions and Answers About Health, Fat and Your Diet

Dietary fat is one of the most controversial and misunderstood subjects in modern nutrition. The following series of questions and answers should help dispel some of the myths and unveil some of the surprising facts about the links between dietary fats and good health.

What types of fat are there?

There are several types of fat, including cholesterol and triglycerides. The latter is the most common form of fat found in animals; it also is found in nuts and seeds, where it serves as stored energy. Triglycerides are simple substances consisting of only four molecules: one is an oily substance, called glycerol, while the other three molecules are substances called fatty acids. These are not acidic in the same way that vinegar or lemon juice are acidic. In this case, the word 'acid' refers to a special combination of atoms at one end of each molecule.

All fatty acids are chains of carbon atoms: some are very short (for example, many of those found in butter) and some carbon chains are very long, containing 20 or even more carbon atoms. Some fatty acid carbon chains are complete and have no spaces for other atoms to join them (*saturated* fatty acids), while others have spaces between carbons where atoms can be added (*unsaturated* fatty acids). The locations on the carbon chain where these unsaturated places between atoms exist are called double-bonds, because neighbouring carbon atoms form a double link to fill the void caused by the missing atom. Double-bonds are unstable and can be damaged by many conditions, including heat and the prescence of free radicals. Almost all of the fats found in beef and lamb are saturated; those predominant in most oils are unsaturated, making them vulnerable to heat and free radicals caused by exposure to the atmosphere and light.

Is fat part of a healthy body?

Yes. Fat is:

- an excellent, compact energy store
- a blanket under the skin that preserves body heat
- a cushion for delicate parts of the body (for example, pads of fat hold the kidneys in place and, within the bony structure of the skull, our eyes are given protective support by fat)
- a part of the structure of every living cell (this is critical to both the form and function of organs in the body and can represent a considerable proportion of their weight; for example, 60 per cent of a normal brain is fat).

Is fat necessary in a healthy diet?

Yes! In a report published in 1994, a panel of experts from the World Health Organization and the Food and Agriculture Organization (WHO/FAO), both agencies of the United Nations, concluded that an adequate amount of dietary fat is essential for health. This quantity must be sufficient to meet energy needs and provide amounts of vitamins and essential fatty acids necessary for normal growth and health.*

* *Fats and Oils in Human Nutrition: Report of a Joint Expert Consultation:* FAO food and nutrition paper (ISBN 92–5–103621–7, WHO/FAO, 1994), available from UNIPUB, 4611F Assembly Drive, Lanham, MD 20706–4391, USA. (A summary of this report is available in *Nutrition Reviews,* Vol. 33, No. 7, pp 202–205, 1995.)

Is there a link between certain kinds of fat and good health?

Yes. Research shows that there is a link between lower levels of risk from major degenerative illnesses, such as heart disease, cancer and arthritis, and diets rich in unsaturated fats, fibre, complex carbohydrates and natural antioxidants. The Mediterranean diet is an example of such a diet. Like many other healthy diets, seed and nut oils are important sources of dietary fat. Everyone should make sure their diet contains these foods.

But don't we eat too much fat?

For many people, the answer is yes. On average, for people in affluent, Western societies the percentage of calories they consume in the form of fat is too high. Without adequate exercise, this may lead to obesity and certain related conditions, including heart disease, stroke and diabetes. For many – but not all – the total amount of fat they eat should be reduced for good health.

However, people on low-calorie diets and active women of child-bearing age may need to increase the amount of polyunsaturated fats they eat.

If the body makes fat from the extra calories we eat, why do we need fat in our food?

During digestion, fats in foods perform certain functions other nutrients cannot. They:

- aid the absorption of fat-soluble vitamins A, D, E and K
- aid in the creation of bile salts, which are needed for digestion
- provide a daily source of essential fatty acids – the special substances the body cannot manufacture from other nutrients.

Are some fats healthier than others?

Yes. Most people eat too much saturated animal fat and not enough polyunsaturated fat, like that in seeds, nuts and vegetable oils. For good health, the dietary balance between oils and saturated fats should be tipped in favour of the oils.

How much fat should we eat each day?

This depends on age, sex and activity level. According to WHO/FAO, for healthy men and older women leading normally active lives, *at least* 15 per cent of the calories they eat should come from fat. Therefore, if an active person requires a daily average of 3,000 calories to meet their energy needs, *at least* 415 of those calories should be fat. Because 1 gram of pure fat contains approximately 9 calories, 50 grams of fat are needed to meet this minimum requirement. (If you have a kitchen scale, measure 50 grams of oil and see how much that is!)

Keep in mind that the word 'fat' is general – it includes saturated, monounsaturated and polyunsaturated fats. Fresh, high-quality oils containing monounsaturated and polyunsaturated fats should provide most of the fat you consume. For good health, no more than 10 per cent of the total calories you consume each day should come from saturated fat.

How much polyunsaturated fat, like that found in oils, should I consume each day?

Based on WHO/ FAO recommendations, an ideal diet contains between 4 and 10 per cent linoleic acid – the type of polyunsaturated fat found in most cooking oils. If you have high cholesterol levels or if you eat large quantities of saturated fat, you should try for the high end of this recommended amount. (But remember, 1 gram of oil does not represent 1 gram of polyunsaturated fat: olive oil contains less than 12 per cent polyunsaturates and in safflower oil the level is above 72 per cent. The percentages of polyunsaturated and other fats found in certain oils, given in *A Directory of Cooking Oils*, page 135, show how widely the proportions of saturated, monounsaturated and polyunsaturated fats can vary.)

Do active young men need to eat proportionally more fat than women of the same age?

No, it is the other way round! During their reproductive years, women need to consume *at least 20 per cent* of their calories as fat. Polyunsaturated oils from seeds, nuts and grains – all of which are rich in essential fatty acids – are good choices for filling this requirement. Everyone needs essential fatty acids in their diet, but pregnant and nursing mothers need to consume enough to meet their own and their children's nutritional requirements.

How much fat do children need in their diet?

This depends on the child's age, but adequate quantities of fat are needed for energy and growth. No child under two years of age should be placed on a low-fat diet and the fats they eat should be rich in polyunsaturated oils, because these are the best source of key essential fatty acids.

In infants, both the amount and type of dietary fat consumed affect growth and development. Breast milk – which contains between 50 and 60 per cent fat – is rich in arachidonic acid (an omega–6 essential fatty acid) and DHA (an omega–3 essential fatty acid). When foods other than breast milk are used to feed infants, care should be taken to ensure that ample levels of these essential fatty acids are present.

During weaning from milk to solids, the fat content of a child's diet should not fall too fast or to too low a level. The WHO/FAO report suggests supplementing the diet of weanlings and infants with vegetable oils to supply necessary fatty acids and maintain the level of calories needed for growth. For children under the age of two, it is recommended that fat should provide between 30 and 40 per cent of the calories in a child's diet, and that the level of essential fatty acids remains similar to those found in breast milk.

What are essential fatty acids?

These are fat molecules the body must have to function normally, but cannot manufacture for itself. They are all polyunsaturated oils. Specific examples are: linoleic acid (found in abundance in oils from various seeds, nuts and grains), gamma-linolenic acid (found in certain flower seeds, such as evening primrose and starflower), alpha-linolenic acid (found in fish, oats and certain grasses and green, leafy vegetables) and DHA and EPA (rich supplies of which are found in fish oil). Essential fatty acids perform the following vital functions in the human body:

- they act as building blocks in the hormone-like substances that regulate many of the body's functions (prostaglandins are one type of substance in this group – prostaglandins are small hormone-like molecules that act as messengers between cells and help regulate many bodily functions, including menstruation and childbirth)
- they help transport cholesterol around the body
- they form part of the structure of normal cell membranes
- they take part in normal cell activities.

All fatty acids are long chains of carbon atoms, each able to 'hook', or 'link', onto four other atoms. In saturated fats, all of these hooks are firmly linked to other atoms. In monounsaturated and polyunsaturated fats, some of these linkages are incomplete and two carbons, located side by side in the chain, form not one but two links with each other. This is called a double-bond. Monounsaturated fats contain one double-bond; polyunsaturated fats two or more. A double-bond is a biologically active area on a fatty acid's carbon chain and its location is critical to how it is used in the body. All essential fatty acids are polyunsaturated and they have a primary – or distinguishing – double-bond either three carbons from the end or six carbons from the end of the carbon chain. These are therefore described as omega–3 and omega–6 fatty acids respectively. Fatty acids with these characteristics cannot be produced in the body and must be obtained from the fats and oils in your diet.

If the body's supply of essential fatty acids is low or slightly deficient, it will try to make substitute molecules. These do not function as needed. Although scientists are still trying to understand the reasons low levels of essential fatty acids probably contribute to the development of certain degenerative illnesses, including heart disease, certain forms of arthritis and some forms of cancer.

What is the medical significance of essential fatty acids in adults?

Many medical scientists believe that if the body's level of essential fatty acids is low for a long period of time, the way is clear for the development of certain major illnesses. These illnesses may develop in several ways: there may be a failure in the system that transports cholesterol around the body or a slowdown in the rate at which certain cells move from place to place. However, one of the most interesting possible effects of low essential fatty acid levels involves the body's ability to produce adequate supplies of special 'messenger' molecules, which help control the body's responses to both internal and external change. For example, prostaglandins are 'messenger' molecules involved in body activities as diverse as giving birth and tissue swelling following a bee sting. Mistakes in the structure of these messengers can result from inadequate supplies of essential fatty acids. These 'crippled' or 'damaged' messengers may be at the root of degenerative illnesses as diverse as cancer, heart disease, kidney disease and the nerve damage which results from diabetes. There is even good reason to believe that essential fatty acids have a role to play in the treatment of certain symptoms of dyslexia.

When are essential fatty acids most important for women?

When they plan to conceive, during pregnancy and while breastfeeding. Expectant and nursing mothers should make sure that their diet contains adequate quantities of oily fish and vegetable oils high in essential fatty acids. Medical scientists estimate that 2.2 grams of essential fatty acids are deposited per day in maternal and foetal tissues during pregnancy.

Why is oily fish important?

In recent years, medical scientists have found that oily fish is rich in substances that appear to protect against heart disease. These are the omega–3 essential fatty acids (also known as n–3 fatty acids). For example, population studies on Eskimos – for whom oily fish is the central food in their diet – have found that they have very low rates of coronary disease.

You can take advantage of the protective effect of omega–3 fatty acids by eating more oily fish, such as mackerel, herring and salmon. Fish oil is particularly high in EPA (eicosapentaenoic acid) and DHA (docosahexaenoic acid). These are the fatty acids needed for the normal development of the human brain and nervous tissue.

Should I consume more omega–6 or omega–3 fatty acids?

According to the joint WHO/FAO report, the ratio of linoleic acid to alpha-linolenic acid in the total fat you eat should be between 5:1 and 10:1. Despite the attention given by the press to the Eskimo diet and omega–3 fatty acids, our bodies actually need significantly more omega–6 fatty acids (derived from the linoleic acid found in most seed and nut oils) than alpha-linolenic acid (found in walnut oil, oily fish, pulses [legumes] and green leafy vegetables). Nevertheless, people consuming a ratio of fatty acids higher than 10:1 should increase the amount of alpha-linolenic acid they consume by either increasing their intake through dietary changes – eating more oily fish, for example – or taking dietary supplements.

Is there a link between antioxidants and dietary fat?

Yes. Considerable excitement has been generated by numerous large research projects linking vitamin E, vitamin C and beta-carotene to reduced levels of certain illnesses. They all appear to block the damage done by dangerous chemical substances known as free radicals.

Although free radicals break down, or destroy, the effectiveness of many necessary substances in the body, they do particular damage to the delicate double-bonds in essential fatty acids. Foods rich in vitamin C – tomatoes, red peppers, strawberries and citrus fruits, for example – and foods rich in vitamin E – especially seeds, nuts and unrefined oils – help stop the action of free radicals.

Aren't people obese because they eat too much fat?

Obesity – excessive amounts of stored body fat – is the visible result of eating more calories than are burned off during normal activity. As all foods contain calories, too much of anything can cause an individual to gain weight. Because the caloric value of fats is more 'dense' than that of carbohydrates and proteins – that is, fats contain approximately twice the number of calories per gram weight as carbohydrates and proteins – fats receive the greatest amount of attention from dietitians and medical professionals. However, it is possible to eat foods containing only carbohydrates and proteins and still gain weight. The secret of weight control is therefore to be found in balancing the number of calories you eat and the number you burn off through activity.

Don't obesity and dietary fats cause disease?

Neither obesity nor dietary fats directly cause disease, although both have been firmly linked with serious illnesses, including certain forms of cancer and heart disease. However, the exact nature of these linkages is unclear and complex.

Over the years, evidence from massive numbers of scientific studies has shown that risk from these diseases may vary with the amount and types of fat eaten, activity levels, quantities of antioxidants consumed, levels of dietary cholesterol and the percentage of total energy that is consumed as fat.

What if I want to eat a low-fat diet to maintain my weight?

As long as you consume enough fat to provide the amount of essential fatty acids and fat-soluble vitamins required for good health and consume enough calories to meet your energy needs, there is no reason to consume more than the levels of fat recommended by WHO/FAO. Cooking with oils is the best way to achieve this goal.

Are there any upper limits to the amount of fat I should eat?

Yes. *Fat should make up no more than 35 per cent of the total calories consumed each day by an active person; people in sedentary jobs, or who are at home most of the time, should limit their intake to 30 per cent.* Putting that in practical terms, an active young man eating a diet containing 3,000 calories a day should consume no more than 1,050 of these calories in the form of fat. Translating calories into weight, that means he should not eat more than 117 grams of fat each day. That is a lot of fat, but have you seen how easy it is to eat a steak and chips (fries) or a Sunday morning fry-up? Both are loaded with fat. Cheddar cheese is about one third fat.

Remember, not all fats are the same. Eat foods high in monounsaturated and polyunsaturated fats. *For good health, limit the saturated fats in your diet to no more than 10 per cent of the total calories you consume.*

Why should I avoid saturated fats?

The links between diet and disease have been the subject of medical research for decades. Although there is still room for considerable debate over many issues, we now feel certain that:

- people who are too fat are prone to developing heart disease, stroke and certain forms of cancer
- high levels of fat in the diet lead to weight gain
- saturated fats – and specifically the animal fats, including butter, lard and tallow – do not contain essential fatty acids
- high levels of saturated fats in the diet have been linked with the development of high cholesterol, arteriosclerosis, heart disease, stroke and cancer.

In other words, eating foods high in saturated fats does little more than provide a compact source of energy. If you are a mountain climber and need a quick energy boost, pull a chocolate bar from your rucksack and go for it. If you sit at your desk most of the day and stare at a word processor, however, think twice before even pulling open the wrapper.

Saturated fats in foods sneak up on you. It is not just the butter on your toast at breakfast that adds weight, it is the fat added to processed foods, which you cannot see, that does the real damage to your waistline.

How much essential fatty acids should I eat?

You should aim to eat foods rich in both linoleic acid and alpha-linolenic acid. *The WHO/FAO report recommends consuming between 4 and 10 per cent of your daily calories as linoleic acid.*

For good health, a woman in her reproductive years should consume more than 20 per cent of calories in the form of fat and up to half of that amount should be from the essential omega–6 fat, linoleic acid.

I don't like using oil. What about margarine made with safflower and sunflower seed oils?

Glance at a bottle of sunflower oil and a tub of sunflower oil margarine and the difference is obvious: one is a fluid, the other is a solid. To be transformed from a light liquid into a spreadable margarine, sunflower oil must go through a series of processes that either destroy most of its delicate double-bonds or bend them around to form *trans*-fats. Scientists have not yet established any relationship between *trans*-fats and illness, but we do know that the body employs them as it would saturated fats and cannot make use of their altered double-bonds.

Margarine was first made as a cheap substitute for butter. Butter has a unique flavour and cooking characteristics that no other fat can match. Each person must make their own choice in these things, but it is not unreasonable to continue to use very modest amounts of butter where its presence makes a significant difference and oils in as many other dishes as possible.

Which oils should I choose for healthy eating?

The fatty acid composition of oils varies greatly, so take nothing for granted. Coconut oil, for example, is rich in saturated fats, although on packaging it is often lumped into the 'vegetable oil' category. When a food's label claims it is rich in vegetable oils, many people assume that means it is rich in polyunsaturated fats and, therefore, good for them. That may not be the case. Unfortunately, coconut oil is popular among food manufacturers because it produces a soothing, smooth, cool feeling in the mouth.

Olive oil is another confusing food. It is a monounsaturated oil, rich in oleic acid, and contains very modest amounts of polyunsaturated linoleic acid.

To help sort out which oil is which, more details on the fat content and cooking characteristics of some oils are provided in *A Directory of Cooking Oils*, page 135.

What are the golden rules for a healthy diet?

- Where possible, substitute foods made and cooked with oils for those prepared with solid fats, like butter and lard.
- Include as many vegetables and fruits as possible. These are rich in the vitamins and minerals you need for health and contain natural antioxidants that help fight the damaging effects of free radicals.
- Use oils when they are fresh. Do not damage the delicate polyunsaturated fats by exposing the oils to too much heat, too much sunlight or too many weeks or months on the shelf after their container has been opened.
- Along with omega–6-rich foods, enjoy cooking ingredients rich in omega–3 fatty acids – such as oily fish, oats and barley.

An important point. People choosing foods rich in saturated fats should aim to include more polyunsaturated oils – rich in linoleic acid – in the foods they eat. If you enjoy sausages and fried bread for breakfast, for example, make sure lunch is based on a salad dressed with a light oil vinaigrette.

Remember, a polyunsaturated oil – sunflower, for example – contains fatty acids other than linoleic. Therefore, 1 gram of oil does not equal 1 gram of linoleic acid.

A Cook's Glossary

antioxidants	natural or synthetic substances that block the damaging effects of free radicals (oxidation) on oils and other substances. Most unrefined oils contain significant quantities of vitamin E, a powerful natural antioxidant. See also *vitamin C* and *vitamin E.*
arugula	see *rocket.*
badiane	see *star anise.*
bake	cook by means of dry heat; little or no fat is needed.
balsamic vinegar	the most exceptional of all vinegars, recognized by its sweet-sour flavour and thick, dark brown appearance. Made only in the area around Modena, Italy, balsamic vinegar is created from concentrated grape juice that is reduced over low heat and then fermented in wooden barrels. There are two grades: industrially produced, which is rather acidic and may have minimal character, and *naturale*, which is made by local families – much the same as fine wines. *Naturale* vinegars require at least 15 years to come to full bloom, but, as vinegars this old are very costly, in the recipes in this book it is suggested that you use vinegars as young as two years. While the price of a bottle of fine balsamic vinegar rivals that of a fine, aged whisky – or more – it is worth the price. Only a few drops are needed to add significant character to a dish. Do not be fooled by cheaper young or blended

products – they will not give a good result.

barbecue cooking on a grill or spit over heat from hot coals, usually outdoors. Barbecued foods are best when kept moist by brushing with a sauce or marinade; oil in these mixtures helps cook the food by holding the heat. Using a Japanese technique, food can be barbecued indoors at the table on a hibachi.

beignet a French word for fritter or doughnut.

beta-carotene a powerful antioxidant found in green, red and yellow vegetables. Beta-carotene has been shown to block the harmful effects of free radicals. Scientific studies suggest it helps prevent cataracts in the eyes and certain other conditions associated with the processes of ageing. It is a precursor of vitamin A, which is not a powerful antioxidant.

blanching cooking herbs and vegetables for a very short time in boiling water. This is useful when you want to preserve the natural colour and texture of leafy greens and for removing the skins from tomatoes, peaches and other fruits.

boil cook by placing food in a fluid, the temperature of which has been raised to its boiling point. While we most often think of boiling in water, oil, and even honey, can be used as cooking media. Boiling in water adds no calories or fat to foods, but may reduce some of their nutritional value and distort their natural colour and texture.

braising cook with very little liquid in a closed pot or pan at a low heat for a long time.

broiling the American term for cooking under a hot grill. See also *grill*.

caramelize browning sugar by melting over a gentle heat. As the sugar changes colour, it loses sweetness and acquires a slightly burnt taste.

carpaccio a way of preparing very thin slices of raw, firm fish or beef in a cold vinaigrette sauce. The dish originated in Italy and is usually served as a starter.

celeriac (celery root) a winter root vegetable popular in France and other West European countries that is delicious shredded and eaten raw in salad or boiled and mashed. Celeriac is low in

	calories and an excellent source of potassium.
celery root	see *celeriac.*
ceps	full-flavoured family of mushroom varieties that have been popular in Europe since the eighteenth century. Like other wild mushrooms prized for their fine flavour, ceps are now cultivated and quite widely available.
clingfilm	plastic wrap used to cover food. Choose a film free of PVC, because it may present a health risk. The packaging will tell you whether or not PVC is present.
Colonna granverde	a fine Italian olive oil in which whole, untreated lemons are included in the processing. The resulting flavour is like no other – densely olive-flavoured, but with a sparkling 'kick' that can only come from the finest, sun-ripened lemons.
confit	an ancient way of preserving meat – especially duck, goose and pork – in which the flesh is slow-cooked in its own fat. After cooking until tender, the meat is then stored in the same fat. Confit is delicious hot or cold. As goose and duck fat are high in monounsaturated fats and as all of the fat should be removed from the meat before serving, confit is relatively low in saturated fats.
curly endive	see frisée.
dice	to cut root vegetables into cubes of a consistent size. Dice may be small or large, but should all be approximately the same size when combined in a recipe. When care is taken in their preparation, dice add considerably to the appearance of a dish.
diet	a combination of all foods and liquids consumed over a period of time. A term most often used in the context of health and healthy eating, diets can be good or bad, heavy or light, vegan or laden with meat. Prescribed diets are selections of foods that are limited for therapeutic purposes.
double-bond	a space between two carbon atoms in a fatty acid that could accept another atom. To fill the place of the missing atom, the two neighbouring carbon atoms form two links, or bonds, between themselves. These are the points of *unsaturation* in the fatty acid, and can be locations for biological

activity. Saturated fats do not contain double-bonds and therefore are not capable of the same kinds of biological activity. See also *saturated fats, monounsaturated fats, polyunsaturated fats, essential fatty acids.*

emulsion — a combination of oil and another fluid in which the two are evenly dispersed for a period of time. Shaking oil and vinegar together results in an emulsion for a minute or two, while adding an emulsifier – an egg yolk, for example – maintains the dispersion for a much longer time. Mayonnaise is an example of an emulsion.

erucic acid — a natural digestive irritant occurring in certain varieties of rapeseed oil (canola). At one time, this was a problem in cattle feed, but now plants grown to produce the seeds used in the commercial preparation of rapeseed oil have been genetically selected to avoid this problem.

essential fatty acids — forms of fat molecules with two or more double-bonds in their carbon chain. These fats are necessary for normal growth and good health. They cannot be manufactured in the human body from other nutrients. There are two types, named for the location of the first double-bonds in the carbon chain: omega–6 fatty acids and omega–3 fatty acids. Linoleic acid, found in rich supply in the oils from nuts and seeds, is the most common form of omega–6 essential fatty acid. Alpha-linolenic acid, the key omega–3 fatty acid, is found in grasses, cows' milk (because they eat grass) and some nuts and seeds but is most highly concentrated in the oil from certain fish. Because these are polyunsaturated fats, their biological activity can be destroyed by heat, free radicals and oxidation. See also *oxidation.*

essential oils — products from plants that carry the distinctive aroma and flavour of the plant. These are not true oils, but another type of substance known as terpenes. Essential oils are soluble in true oils and are used in different concentrations for cooking and aromatherapy.

fats — the high-energy natural components of living materials. All organisms need fat to maintain their natural structure and function. Most fat is in the form of triglycerides, which consist of three long-chain molecules, known as fatty acids, and a molecule of glycerol. Triglycerides make up the majority of fats in both animals in plants. Waxes, phospholipids and cholesterol are also types of fat. See also *oils, saturated fats, monousaturated fats and polyunsaturated fats.*

free radicals — rogue molecules that damage other molecules by destroying their natural electrical balance. Free radicals are part of many normal life processes, but, in abnormally large numbers, they cause damage that leads to cell death and disease. Unsaturated fatty acids, especially polyunsaturated essential fatty acids, are easily damaged by free radicals. See *antioxidants.*

frisée (curly endive) — a good salad vegetable. The outer green leaves can be bitter, so, for most salads, use only the inner yellow heart. This and similar salad ingredients lift or add height to a plate of food and greatly enhance its appearance.

fry — cook by means of heating a thin layer of food in a layer of hot fat (butter, oil, lard) in a shallow pan. Once cooked, fried foods should be drained on paper kitchen towel because they tend to absorb considerable amounts of the fat they were cooked in, which adds calories and increases the daily quantity of fat consumed. Deep frying involves immersing food completely in very hot fat. Again, drain food to remove the excess fat before serving. Many foods are fried at very high temperatures, which may cause smoking and damage the nutritional value of delicate polyunsaturated oils.

grill (broil) — a method of rapid cooking that seals food by exposing it to the radiant heat from charcoal, gas or an electric bar. Oil-based marinades are often used to help seal the food.

infusion — the process of capturing the aroma and flavour of a herb or spice by letting it steep in a fluid. Milk can be infused with vanilla, wine with cinnamon and cloves, oil with truffle and garlic. Some foods do not give up their character easily during infusion, so gentle heating aids the process. Tea is a good example of a hot infusion.

Jerusalem artichoke — a root vegetable, or tuber, that originates from North America and was introduced into Europe by Champlain.

The taste resembles that of true artichokes – thus the name – but the two plants are totally different. Jerusalem artichoke tubers can be very knobbly and difficult to peel. If they are, try blanching them first.

julienne — food cut into very thin strips using a sharp knife or mandoline. For vegetables, pieces cut 5 mm (¼ in) thick and 2.5 cm (1 in) long are ideal. See also *mandoline*.

linoleic acid — an omega–6 essential fatty acid found in polyunsaturated oils from seeds and nuts. During metabolism, linoleic acid is transformed into gamma-linolenic acid (GLA). See also *essential fatty acids*.

lollo rosso — round, very curly lettuce with purple-red streaks on bright green leaves; good for adding texture and height to a dish.

mandoline — a two-part slicer with a range of cutting surfaces that is particularly useful when preparing thin, even pieces of apples, cabbage, potatoes and other root vegetables. Made properly, slices prepared using a mandoline add an attractive, professional appearance to food. If you are investing in one, buy the best you can afford as, cleaned and stored properly, a good-quality mandoline will give years of service.

marinade — a mixture in which meats and fish are steeped to infuse them with flavour or tenderize them prior to cooking. See also *marinate*.

marinate — the process of steeping fish, poultry, meat and sometimes fruit in a marinade. See also *marinade*.

mille-feuille — a French culinary term for a dish made of fine, crisp pastry layered with cream, jam or fruit. Traditionally, the pastry used for *mille-feuille* is made with a considerable quantity of butter. In this book, a recipe is given that uses a modest quantity of oil to make biscuits (cookies) for assembling into *mille-feuille*-like desserts (see page 111).

mirepoix — finely diced vegetables used to enhance the flavour of a sauce or braised dish. Standard ingredients are onions, celery and carrots – a magic combination of tastes.

monounsaturated fats — the dominant type of fat found in duck fat, olive oil and

	avocados. Credited by many with the ability to lower blood cholesterol levels, each molecule of monunsaturated fats contains only one double-bond. This makes them less susceptible to damage from exposure to heat and oxygen than are the more delicate polyunsaturated fats. See also *double-bond.*
nappage	a French culinary term for a sauce or dressing that is made to cover a dish. Poached fish is sometimes served with a *nappage.*
non-stick pan	a modern cooking utensil lined with a special coating that avoids food sticking, thus reducing the amount of fat needed for frying. The coating in some pans is affected by very high heat and so should be used only at lower temperatures. When selecting non-stick pans, choose those that can be used at normal frying temperatures. See also *fry.*
nutrition	the balanced combination of foods supplying the body with all of the substances (nutrients) it needs for normal growth and good health.
oils	types of fat that are fluid at room temperature because they are rich in polyunsaturated and monounsaturated fatty acids. Margarine, a firmer form of fat, is made from oils by reducing the unsaturated structure of their molecules.
oxidation	damage caused by exposing food and other substances to the air. Oxygen in the air interacts with other molecules and causes foods to become rancid, resulting in a wholly unpleasant taste and odour. Free radicals are involved in the oxidation process and natural antioxidants, such as vitamin E, help slow its progress. The double-bonds in oils are highly susceptible to oxidation, making it necessary to protect polyunsaturated oils from excessive heat and air and light. See *double-bond* and *rancid.*
plastic wrap	see *clingfilm.*
polyunsaturated fats	fats – always fluid – in which the majority of the molecules contain at least two double-bonds. Linoleic acid, the key omega–6 fatty acid, is a major constituent in polyunsaturated oils in seeds and most nuts and is required for normal growth and good health. Because double-bonds are fragile

and are destroyed by high heat, sunlight and air, polyunsaturated oils need to be kept in capped containers on cool, dark shelves in the kitchen. These oils are not suitable for deep frying at high temperatures.

poulet noire — a fine-quality free-range French chicken raised on a diet of grains and maize (corn).

rancid — fats and oils exposed to heat, light and air soon develop an unpleasant smell and flavour because they have become oxidized. In this process, oxygen combines with the unsaturated fatty acids and damages their natural structure, robbing them of much of their nutritional value. Once a bottle of delicate, unrefined polyunsaturated oil is opened, it must be capped and placed in a cool, dark place to prevent it becoming oxidized, or rancid.

reduction — a thickened sauce with a highly concentrated flavour, made by evaporating off, or reducing, the volume of a fluid in the mixture by boiling.

refined oil — any oil from a plant source that has been treated to remove unwanted colour, flavour or sediment. Refined oils keep for longer periods of time than unrefined oils and can be used for cooking at higher temperatures, but do not have the same flavour strength. Extra virgin olive oil purchased in an unrefined state may contain some sediment.

refresh — to rapidly cool blanched food by running cold water over it. This stops the cooking process and helps retain the food's crispness and colour.

render (fat) — to 'melt' – or release – fat from poultry or meat by cooking. Chicken fat can be rendered by placing pads of fat from a fresh bird in a small pan of water and simmering for 20–30 minutes. The oily fat will be released from the tissue into the water, from which it can be separated after cooling.

roast see *bake* — to help seal in their natural juices and prevent drying, vegetables are best when brushed with oil before roasting.

rocket (arugula) — a leafy green plant, popular among Mediterranean cooks, which has a distinctive, pungent taste and aroma. Use only small, young leaves for salads and sauces as the older leaves have a strong mustard taste.

saffron	the dried stigmas from the flowers of the saffron crocus. As the stigmas are picked by hand, and 25 g (1 oz) of the spice contains many thousands of stigmas, saffron is expensive. However, its fine yellow colour and unique flavour make it worth the cost. Try the infusion recipe included in this book (see page 14) to help get the greatest value from a small amount of spice. Also, add the saffron near the end of the cooking process to preserve its flavour and do not put saffron directly into a pan in which you are frying food.
saturated fats	fats containing no double-bonds. Fats from beef and sheep, butter and cheese are highly saturated. In contrast to oils and other fats containing large amounts of polyunsaturated fatty acids, which are fluid in cool temperatures, saturated fats are hard in such temperatures. Research has shown that people eating large amounts of saturated fats in their diets over time have a greater risk of developing heart disease and certain forms of cancer than those who consume moderate amounts of these fats.
sauté	to cook food in fat in a frying pan until browned. As sautéd foods tend to absorb fat, it is healthier to use oils than butter or animal fat.
sea salt	salt obtained by evaporating seawater. Because it is high in many minerals, such as potassium and magnesium, and full of a real 'salty' flavour, modest amounts of sea salt add flavour and nutritional value to food without pushing up the sodium content. Although sea salt seems expensive, it is well worth the cost. Among the best is that from Maldon, in Essex, England, and western France, where it is called *la fleur de sel*, or the flower of the salt (my favourite is *sel de Guérande*, from the western Loire region).
shiitake mushrooms	an oriental mushroom cultivated in many parts of the world and valued for its meaty texture and flavour. Absolutely delicious fried in olive oil with a little garlic, salt and pepper!
simmer	to heat and maintain a fluid at a temperature just below boiling point. If you watch a simmering pan, the surface of the liquid will move slightly, and now and again a bubble will come to the surface.

smoke point — the temperature at which the molecules in a cooking fat begin to break down and form smoke. Foods cooking when the smoke point is reached are often ruined. Smoke points vary depending on the type of fat. Saturated fats – clarified butter, for example – have high smoke points, while those for oils are much lower, and decrease as the percentage of polyunsaturates increases. Therefore, refined olive oil is a good medium for frying, while safflower and sunflower oils are not. Never try to fry with walnut oil.

star anise — an ancient spice that looks like an eight-pointed star and tastes a little like aniseed. The flavour is hot and makes a nice contrast with fatty fish and poultry. This makes it a popular ingredient with cooks from Scandinavia to China.

stir-fry — a quick cooking method best done in a round-bottomed oriental wok over a high heat. As only a small amount of oil is used, this is a low-fat way to prepare food.

stock — a broth prepared by cooking vegetables, herbs and, often, meat or bones in plenty of water over a low heat for a long time.

tapenade — a condiment originally from Provence, France, containing anchovies, olives and capers. The name comes from the Provençal word for capers, *tapeno*.

vinegar — an ancient cooking ingredient made by fermenting wine or other fruit juice. Fermentation gives vinegar its sharp taste. See also *balsamic vinegar*.

vitamin C — a powerful natural antioxidant found in citrus fruit, strawberries and other plants that protects against oxidation by free radicals in watery fluids.

vitamin E — a powerful natural antioxidant found in nut and seed oils that helps prevent oxidation by free radicals. Wheatgerm oil is a rich source of vitamin E.

zest — the oily, highly scented and coloured outer rind of citrus fruit. When used in cooking, the zest must be separated from the white, inner part of the skin – the pith – as it has a bitter taste. Zest can be removed with either a sharp knife or a gadget called a zester, which cuts a very shallow strip from the rind.

A Directory of Cooking Oils

Selecting oils for cooking at home is very much a matter of individual preference. For example, some people are passionate about the flavour of unrefined groundnut oil (peanut oil) and sherry vinegar on cold vegetable salad, while others find the idea revolting. There are no right or wrong choices. However, if you have never cooked with a *range* of oils before, it is difficult to know where to begin. Chapter 1 contains some good tips on tasting and trying oils. In addition, the following list of speciality oils and their characteristics should help you select one or two to get you started on building a collection of oils you like to use.

Considerable confusion surrounds the terms used to describe oils. To help dispel the mystery, here are some general guidelines.

Unrefined oils (virgin oils)

These oils have had least done to them. All oils are pressed or extracted by means of heat, pressure or chemicals. Certain oils cannot be used without harsh processing – cotton seed oil is an example of such an oil. However, other oils – olive and nut oils are good examples – have the strongest flavour and most appealing colour when processing is as gentle and minimal as possible. Just remember that unrefined oils often have residue in them. That is why you may see a dark brown sediment in the bottom of the bottle of some of the best olive oils. What is more, as not all of the material from the original seeds or nuts has been removed from unrefined oils, they burn, or smoke, at lower temperatures than the refined varieties. This same residual material can contain nutrients, such as vitamin E, which can add to a healthy diet. On the negative side, unrefined oils are expensive, sometimes hard to find and become rancid soon after opening and exposure to air.

Refined oils

These oils are more stable than unrefined oils and can be heated to higher temperatures. They also have the advantage of being easier to locate and less expensive. Good blended vegetable oil, which is highly processed, is excellent for deep frying (just remember to filter it between uses and don't use it more than two or three times, although, this said, fresh is always best).

Using the directory

To help you choose oils for healthy eating, the average fatty acid content of most oils is included in its description below. As you would guess, 'S' indicates the percentage of saturated fats in an oil, 'M' is the percentage of monounsaturated fats and 'P' indicates the percentage of polyunsaturated fats. This information, marked with *, is taken from *McCance and Widdowson's The Composition of Foods,* 5th Edition, and reproduced here with the permission of The Royal Society of Chemistry and the Controller of Her Majesty's Stationery Office.

Unfortunately, such exact figures are not available for all of the oils listed below. Percentage figures given for certain nut oils – hazelnut and walnut, for example – reflect the composition of the oil as found in the nut itself. As an example, in the first entry – almond oil – the figures show a higher level of monounsaturated fats than polyunsaturated fats; the oil contains less than 5 per cent saturated fat.

Oils high in monounsaturates share many of the health benefits associated with olive oil, including a high percentage of the fat known as oleic acid. Oils high in polyunsaturates are rich in linoleic acid – a key essential fatty acid. Walnut oil is a good source of both linoleic – an omega–6 fatty acid – and linolenic acid – an omega–3 fatty acid.

The oils

almond

although expensive, unrefined almond oil is full of the natural, sumptuous character of the taste and aroma of the nut. Golden brown oil from roasted almonds adds significantly to the flavour of salads and dressings for cold meats. But, a word of caution: as is true with all unrefined, or virgin, oils, heating this delicate product destroys its character and even heating it to relatively low temperatures results in smoking and burning.

Oil extracted from almonds and refined has little taste or scent. Pure almond oil can be used to coat the internal surfaces of baking tins, as it will have little effect on the flavour of the final product – unlike butter or margarine, for example. (S 4.7, M 34.4, P 14.2)

avocado — an avocado is the fruit of a tree belonging to the laurel family. Not unlike the fruit of the olive tree, the flesh surrounding the seed is rich in monounsaturated fatty acids. When extracted, avocado oil is a delicious, cream-like base for salad dressings and topping for cold fish, but, be careful, this is a delicate ingredient. Its special characteristics should be protected by refrigeration and it should never be heated. (S 22.3, M 65.7, P 12.0)

Oil is also extracted from the hard avocado stones (pits), but it has little to offer in the way of individual character.

canola — see *rapeseed*.

coconut — this is a highly saturated form of fat and although it has much to offer in terms of its flavour and cooking characteristics, its health benefits are limited to its use as a high energy source. It is a popular choice for commercial sweet (candy) and biscuit (cookie) manufacturers, though, because it gives a pleasant, 'cooling' sensation in the mouth and is often found as one of the 'hidden' fats in the processed foods we eat. (S 85.2, M 6.6, P 1.7*)

colza — see *rapeseed*.

corn (maize) — a deep golden yellow, refined corn oil is one of the most widely used and economical of all oils. Even after refining, it maintains the distinctive taste of corn, making it an interesting choice for baking and deep frying – it adds considerably to the flavour of chips (fries) and batter. For some, the taste is too heavy for salad dressings or mayonnaise. It can be heated to 200°C/390°F for frying.

In some places it is possible to purchase unrefined corn oil, which has an even stronger characteristic flavour. It blends well with root vegetables and light meats, such as chicken. However, like all unrefined oils, it should not be heated to temperatures required for deep frying and is best used in sauces, dressings and for baking. If you enjoy corn on the cob, try brushing one with unrefined corn oil instead of butter before you sprinkle on the salt. (S 12.7, M 24.7, P 57.8*)

cotton seed — this food product originated as a byproduct of the textile industry. When the oil is first extracted from the cotton seeds, it is a dark reddish colour, has a strong scent and is clouded with impurities. However, once processed and bleached, the resulting product is economical and good for cooking. Large quantities are used in the manufacture of commercial food products and much of the oil used is blended and sold as 'vegetable oil' or 'cooking oil'. At one point, there was evidence that some cotton seed oil suffered pesticide contamination, but that is no longer the case and oils sold commercially are safe. More cotton seed oil is used in North America than in Europe. (S 25.6, M 21.3, P 48.1*)

fruit oils — these are not oils, but substances known as 'terpenes'. Also known as essential oils, fruit oils have much to offer as sources of flavour when diluted with true oils.

grapeseed — this oil, extracted from grape pips (seeds), has a wonderful green colour and a delicate, almost neutral flavour. As the cost is reasonable, grapeseed oil is an excellent choice for blending with heavier nut oils, such as hazelnut or walnut, which may be too strong by themselves, and using in sauces and dressings. It is a good choice, too, for marinating meat and, as a refined product, grapeseed oil is an excellent choice for frying because it stands up well to heat. It is also rich in monounsaturated fats.

groundnut (peanut) — highly refined oils extracted from peanuts (groundnuts), are used widely in many parts of the world, from China and Africa to France and America. In this form, the oil has none of the distinctive flavour of the nut, but has a fine texture that makes it suitable not only for frying and baking, but also for blending into dressings, sauces and mayonnaise. A great advantage of this oil is that it can be heated to temperatures up to 175°C/350°F and, when filtered well, can be reused five or six times for deep frying.

In its unrefined form, though, groundnut oil (peanut oil) should never be used at high temperatures. However, it is full of the flavour of the roasted nuts and makes an excellent dressing for meat and root vegetable dishes. When diluted with a neutral oil, it can add a special lift to fried potatoes or other vegetables. (S 18.8, M 47.8, P 28.5*)

hazelnut — this wonderful brown oil is excellent on its own or blended with a fine wine or sherry vinegar to serve drizzled on salads, fish, meats and root vegetables. As hazelnut oil is expensive and susceptible to oxidation after opening, it makes sense to buy small quantities of the best product you can find and use it with abandon while it is still fresh. Oils produced in France are of exceptional quality.

Substituting hazelnut oil for a small portion of the fat in a baking recipe can dramatically enhance the aroma and flavour of the final product. (S 4.7, M 50, P 5.9)

mustard — this name can be used to refer to two very different types of oil. Rapeseed oil (canola) is sometimes referred to as mustard oil because the rapeseed plant is from the same botanical family as the mustard plant and has similar yellow flowers. More correctly, however, the name belongs to the mustard plant itself.

In their delightful book, *The Compleat Mustard,* Rosamond Man and Robin Weir describe the valued place mustard holds in traditional Russian life. The oil is also used, much like the finest olive oil, in homes around the Mediterranean and in India, this distinctively flavoured oil is used in both cooking and as a domestic fuel.

olive — throughout this book, much has been said about the special qualities of olive oil. Quite simply, for many foods, olive oil in its many forms is king. Try sampling oils from the south of France and compare them with oils from fruit grown in Portugal or the United States. As is true of wines, the robustness of flavour, aroma and colour of extra virgin and virgin olive oils are heavily influenced by climate and the land on which the mother-plants are grown. (S 14, M 69.7, P 11.2*)

peanut — see *groundnut*.

pistachio — a dark green, sweetly nutty flavoured product, pistachio oil is excellent as a dressing on foods with dense, meaty tastes, such as duck salad, meat pâté and cold sliced lamb. Good counter-flavours include sherry and balsamic vinegars. Like other fine nut oils, exposure to heat destroys its distinctive flavour and opened bottles should be kept in a cool, dark place.

This is an example of a speciality oil that may be difficult to find. If you see a bottle, swallow hard when you see the price and try some. Like olive oil, it is rich in monounsaturates and goes well with duck, quail, firm white fish and salads. (S 4.1, M 15.2, P 9.8)

pumpkin seed (marrowseed oil) — this oil is difficult to obtain but worth the price. Unrefined pumpkin seed oil carries the musky flavour of the fruit of the plant from which it comes. Dark and thick, much like the oil from sesame seeds, pumpkin seed oil should be kept for dressing salads or hot vegetables or used as part of a blend of ingredients for fish. Avoid high temperatures, as they will destroy the oil and make it bitter.

rapeseed (canola, colza) — the plant from which this seed oil is produced has a culinary history dating back to the Romans. Finding it viable in colder climates, which olive trees are not, Roman battalions carried its tiny seeds north as far as Britain, where today it remains a major source of oil.

High in polyunsaturated fatty acids, this bland-tasting oil is a good choice for most sauces and dressings because it does not compete with the flavour of other ingredients in a dish. However, because the level of polyunsaturates is very high, it is not a good choice for deep frying. If it is your choice for frying, use it only once or twice and filter it between times.

Certain varieties of rapeseed are high in eruic acid,

a substance known to cause tissue damage in animals. However, through bioengineering and plant-breeding programmes, the level of this irritant has been substantially reduced. In fact, refined rapeseed oil (canola) has gained wide popularity among food manufacturers and consumers alike and may become one of the dominant oils during the twenty-first century. (Oil from seeds low in eruic acid contains: S 6.6, M 57.2, P 31.5*)

rice bran — this oil is difficult to obtain for home use. In an unrefined state, its characteristics are similar to those of wheatgerm oil.

safflower — this oil is a good choice for dressing salads, baking and grilling (broiling). However, because safflower oil is particularly high in unsaturated fatty acids, especially linoleic acid (75 per cent), the high heats of frying can destroy much of its health value. Safflower oil is also rich in vitamin E, making it a good choice for dressings and sauces.

The benefits of safflower oil have made it popular among health-conscious eaters. Taking advantage of this, some margarine manufacturers have developed products using this oil as a healthy living alternative to butter. However, to convert the liquid oil to a harder, 'spreadable' product, various chemical processes are used that destroy the all-important double-bonds in safflower oil's polyunsaturated fatty acids, thereby lowering the final product's health value. People enjoying the flavour of safflower-based margarine should check the packaging to see if it lists the amount of *trans* fatty acids the hardening processes have created. (S 10.2, M 12.6, P 72.1*)

sesame — exotic images from the Ancient World and Orient are evoked by even a quick whiff of sesame seed oil being tossed with freshly steamed or wok-fried vegetables. A native of Africa, sesame has been grown in China and India for millennia. High in linoleic acid (about 40 per cent), sesame oil is an excellent addition to your kitchen stores. However, its pungent, nutty aroma may be too strong for many dishes and dilution with grapeseed or almond oil may be desirable for some foods.

Several forms of sesame seed oil are available. Highly refined products have little flavour and oxidize slowly. Unrefined oil has the natural, distinctive, nutty flavour of the seeds and is an excellent choice for many baked products. Of all the varieties, unrefined sesame oil has the greatest health benefits, but, because it oxidizes easily, it should be kept in a cool, dark place and consumed quickly.

Oil pressed from roasted seeds has a unique flavour and is highly praised by oriental cooks. One tip: unrefined sesame oil – from either raw or roasted seeds – should not be exposed to high heat, because it burns easily. Use it on vegetables, fish or noodles after they are cooked and just before serving. (S 14.2, M 37.3, P 43.9*)

soya — refined, or processed, oil from soya beans is one of the most widely used food products in the world. Inexpensive and lacking any significant flavour of its own, it is excellent for baking, frying and grilling (broiling). (S 14.5, M 23.2, P 56.5*)

sunflower — in its refined form, moderately priced sunflower oil is high in polyunsaturated fatty acids, neutral in flavour and light in texture. This combination of characteristics makes it an excellent choice for both frying foods and dressing salads. As it has little flavour of its own, it is ideal for making mayonnaise and sauces, which may be flavoured with more expensive, pungent oils.

A word of warning: because sunflower oil is rich in polyunsaturated fats, it is not a good choice for deep frying. (S 11.9, M 20.2, P 63*)

vegetable oil — products labelled 'vegetable oil' are usually blends of highly refined oils (including cotton seed and soya), designed to meet certain temperature and cost limits. As these are highly processed oils, they will withstand the high temperatures needed for deep frying and, for the cook on a budget, these oils are the cheapest to buy. They have no flavour advantage, however. Remember, always filter oils after deep frying and restrict the number of times you reuse a batch of oil. (Average: S 10.4, M 35.5, P 48.2*)

walnut — truly one of the great oils. Heavy with the dark flavours of the nuts from which it is pressed, walnut oil is popular in both France and Italy.

Like many good wines, this oil is prepared in small batches by local producers, making it expensive and adding to the variations in taste and quality available. Some carry the sharp taste of the shell, while others are creamy smooth reflections of the rich meat of the nut. Whichever is your particular favourite, try adding walnut oil to pastry and breads or as a complementary taste in puréed root vegetables. Blended with sherry vinegar or lemon juice, walnut oil makes an excellent sauce for fish or salad.

Walnut oil contains a high proportion of unsaturated fatty acids, but is especially rich in the essential fatty acids, linoleic and linolenic, making it an excellent healthy choice for home cooking. These same constituents, however, make walnut oil highly susceptible to oxidation, so store opened bottles of this fine product in a cool, dark place. (S 5.6, M 12.4, P 47.5)

wheatgerm

this oil is extracted from the heart of the wheat kernel, the germ, and is a very rich source of vitamin E and essential fatty acids. Because this oil is thick and has a rather strong flavour, its utility in everyday cooking is limited. However, it is an excellent food supplement. Once opened, this oil is best kept in the refrigerator. (S 18.8, M 15.9, P 60.7*)

Weight and Measures

Weights

When using or adapting a recipe, do not mix the metric, imperial or American measures as they are not interchangeable.

Metric	Imperial
7 g	¼ oz
15 g	½ oz
22 g	¾ oz
25 g	1 oz
40 g	1½ oz
50 g	2 oz
65 g	2½ oz
75 g	3 oz
100 g	4 oz
150 g	5 oz
175 g	6 oz
200 g	7 oz
225 g	8 oz
250 g	9 oz
275 g	10 oz
300 g	11 oz
350 g	12 oz
375 g	13 oz
400 g	14 oz
425 g	15 oz
450 g	16 oz (1 lb)

Spoon measures

Metric	Imperial
1.25 ml	¼ teaspoon
2.5 ml	½ teaspoon
5 ml	1 teaspoon
7.5 ml	1½ teaspoon
10 ml	2 teaspoons
15 ml	3 teaspoons (1 tablespoon)
30 ml	2 tablespoons

Liquids

Metric	Imperial (American)
25 ml	1 fl oz
40 ml	1½ fl oz
50 ml	2 fl oz (¼ cup)
85 ml	3 fl oz
100 ml	3½ fl oz
120 ml	4 fl oz (½ cup)
150 ml	5 fl oz
250 ml	8 fl oz (1 cup)
275 ml	9 fl oz
300 ml	10 fl oz
350 ml	12 fl oz
375 ml	13 fl oz
400 ml	14 fl oz
450 ml	15 fl oz
475 ml	16 fl oz (1 pint)
600 ml	20 fl oz
1000 ml (1 litre)	1¾ pints

Oven Temperatures

Degrees centigrade	Degrees fahrenheit	Gas
110	225	¼
120	250	½
140	275	1
150	300	2
170	325	3
180	350	4
190	375	5
200	400	6
220	425	7
230	450	8
240	475	9
260	500	10

Bibliography and Further Reading

Coultate, T. P., *Food: The Chemistry of Its Components* (The Royal Society of Chemistry, Cambridge, England, 1989)

Ewin, Jeannette, *The Fats We Need to Eat* (Thorsons, London, England, 1995)

Fats and Oils in Human Nutrition: Report of a Joint Expert Consultation: FAO food and nutrition paper (ISBN 92–5–103621–7, WHO/FAO, 1994), available from UNIPUB, 4611F Assembly Drive, Lanham, MD 20706–4391, USA. (A summary of this report is available in *Nutrition Reviews,* Vol. 33, No. 7, pp 202–205, 1995.)

Lawson, Harry, *Food Oils and Fats: Technology, Utilization and Nutrition* (Chapman and Hall, New York, USA, 1995)

McCance and Widdowson's The Composition of Foods, Fifth Edition (Royal Society of Chemistry and Ministry of Agriculture, Fisheries and Food, Cambridge, England, 1991).

Man, Rosamond, and Weir, Robin, *The Compleat Mustard* (Constance and Company Limited, London, England, 1988)

Index